RIGHT OVER THE MOUNTAIN
Travels with a Tibetan Medicine Man

Gill Marais is a photojournalist who lives and works in Paris. She was born in South Africa, and has travelled extensively in the East and South-East Asia.

RIGHT OVER
THE MOUNTAIN

TRAVELS WITH A
TIBETAN MEDICINE MAN

GILL MARAIS

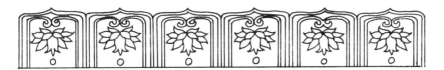

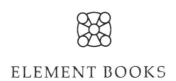

ELEMENT BOOKS

© Gill Marais 1991

First published in France in 1988 by Editions Sand.
First English Edition published in Great Britain in 1991
by Element Books Limited
Longmead, Shaftesbury, Dorset

Cover illustration: *Path to Kailas* by Nicholas Roerich.
Courtesy of the Nicholas Roerich Museum, New York.
Cover design by Max Fairbrother
Designed by Roger Lightfoot
Typeset by BP Integraphics
Printed and bound in Great Britain by
Dotesios Printers Ltd, Trowbridge, Wiltshire

British Library Cataloguing in Publication Data
Marais, Gill
Right over the mountain : travels with a Tibetan medicine man.
1. Asia. Himalayas. Description & travel
I. Title
915.40452

ISBN 1-85230-150-3

CONTENTS

'A Human being is part of the whole. . . . He experiences himself, his thoughts and feelings as something separate from the rest . . . a kind of optical delusion of his consciousness. This delusion is a kind of prison for us, restricting us to our personal desires and to affection for a few persons nearest us. Our task must be to free ourselves from this prison by widening our circle of compassion to embrace all living creatures, and the whole of nature in its beauty. Nobody is able to achieve this completely, but striving for such achievement is, in itself, a part of the liberation and a foundation for inner security.'

Albert Einstein

'Each of us must act as the pilot of his own soul on its solitary voyage throughout the unknown. The loneliness of the individual human soul is one of the saddest facts of human experience. But there are divine moments in the lives of at least some of us when by the contemplation of the extremely beautiful in nature . . . we feel our loneliness is a mere appearance which will pass away: moments in which we feel we will be in communion and fellowship with the perfect beauty and white truth beyond the fleeting shadow land in which we daily move.'

Reginald Flemming Johnson

(Tutor to Pu Yi, the last Emperor of China, in his chronicle *From Peking to Mandalay* written in the early years of this century.)

PROLOGUE

———————— • ————————

*A journey through space and time from Paris
to Kashmir and up into the Zangskar valley—
Ladakh—It prepares us for the Amchi's world*

THROUGH SPACE AND TIME

I grew up in a harsh land where animals and birds survived in sparse vegetation. Each spring, the earth burst into flower carpeting the hills with daisies bright as a rainbow's promise. Bushmen sometimes came out of the desert to work on the farms. They seldom stayed longer than a year before slipping away, silent as shadows, from the mesh of civilisation. I loved those little people with their delicate gestures and their low, gentle voices, and would sit with them on the rocks, intrigued by their tales of magic. They told of a time when a Dream was dreaming us, and in those dream-stories, men, animals and plants spoke together. Harmonious discourse was everywhere.

Once, during a solar eclipse, I watched a tortoise pull in its head and freeze as the moon's shadow raced across the earth. All sound ceased. All life's movement came to a halt, and I was overtaken by a fear of an unknown kind. Was this what it would be like at the end of the world? That acute sensation of vulnerability left me with a profound respect for the forces of nature and the immense power of the sun which had hung black in the sky, its orb surrounded by white flames of terrifying brilliance. My young mind was overwhelmed. For the first time I sensed that all life was interconnected.

Years later, I felt that same awe in the Himalayas. The high desert plateaus slashed by valleys and seemingly planted with mountains, evoked the grandeur of the Africa I had loved as a child. But, in those expanses, instead of Bushmen, lived Buddhists whose

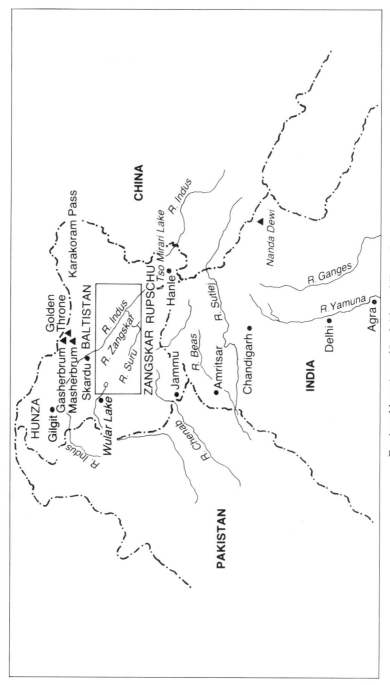

Regional location of Ladakh and Zangskar

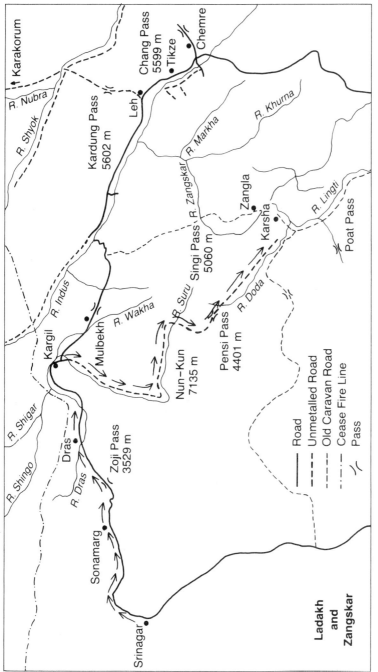

Detail of Ladakh and Zangskar

religion and medicine contained the same holistic view of man. For them, all things are born from the five great Elements of Creation; Earth, Water, Fire, Air and Space. Because of my early environment, such an idea was far from alien to me, I knew it sprang from the Vedic philosophy already flourishing in India 1500 years before Christ. Eastern thought had intrigued me since adolescence.

Now, after the collapse of my marriage, I felt a desperate need to get away from Paris and find healing for that damaged part of myself which was still firmly shackled in the past. The end of my marriage had been bitter, angry and resentful. I had taken refuge in my work as a photojournalist which had left me little time for self-pity or regret. But in those inevitable moments of solitary doubt and fear, I had found solace in my friends. Good friends, warm friends, who were generous in their understanding. People like Alice, deserted by her husband, bedridden with cancer, who yet had the time and kindness of spirit to console others in their pain. I had talked with her of places I had been to and would like to visit again and it was she who had suggested that I dissolve rancid memories in the vast silence of the Himalayas that I had discovered on a journey years before.

Exactly one week later I met John Roberts, a British television producer, at a party. He had just completed a documentary on a Tibetan country doctor, or Amchi, in the Zangskar valley of Ladakh, east of Kashmir. I told him of my plans. 'Why not write an article on Tibetan medicine?' he said, 'Absolutely fascinating. They see energy and matter, spirit and body in quite different perspectives from us.' I would have liked more details but John was already late for a dinner date. As a parting shot, he called out 'He lives in Karsha. Once over the mountain, turn right and ask for Sonam.' I jotted down the name and village on the back of a matchbox. That night, I wrote to Nazir, my Kashmiri friend and guide – the brother I had never had. He replied by telegram: 'Ready for anything at anytime. Love N.' I booked a flight to Delhi and on to Srinagar, the capital of Kashmir, from where we would motor into Ladakh.

While packing, I asked myself what were my secret desires and how I could realise them. I was sure of only one thing. I must find anew a sense of wonder, that 'emerveillement' of nature that had marked my childhood. And, with the focus on Tibetan medicine, what followed time would divulge. I had lost touch with myself. Habit and automatic response had made routine bearable, but they had cast me adrift, alienating me from healing myself. I had grown stale. The inner me slumbered like a child, ignored for too long and told to go away and play while the grown-ups did important things. In most cases, the child within, having gone to sleep, never wakes up, and contact is lost with all that sparkles. We age before our flesh has weakened. Our ego grows touchy and cranky when it should express itself better to all advantage in zest for life; not selfishness. Change of place, they say, changes the attitude. Up till now, I had travelled not to change my ideas but to add more to those already in residence. This time my motives were different. My escape would be an inner journey to the unknown and the unpredictable. In my travels I have always sought a correspondence between places and happenings and the response they evoke within me. Rather than brave the cold turbulence of wild seas or the darkness behind the moon, I had been drawn to the highest of mountains and the grandest of vistas. My search now was for clarity. This time I was to enter the subterranean labyrinth of my being and journey for a while alone.

LINKS WITH THE PAST

The plane swooped off and a parade of pictures turned in my mind. My first vision was of Katmandu, my first experience of the east. The Buddhist temple hung with coloured silks. The smell of rancid butter and stale incense clogged the air. Monks were sipping tea; a homely touch that reminded me that worship involves man in his entirety. A young French doctor introduced me to a Tibetan pharmacy with shelves of dried herbs and powdered minerals. White masked Tibetans rolled ingredients into pellets. It all looked very primitive.

Tibetan cures work slowly. Their secret is balance; balance between the outer and the inner, the body and the mind, the earth and the heavens.

Then my mind turned to Kashmir. My first encounter with Nazir was under a giant chenar tree on a lawn running down to house-boats on a lake adorned with pink water lilies. Abdul, my elderly host, his white turban crisp against apricot skin, reclined in his garden pavilion. His friend, Nazir, an unusual young man, a Muslim educated by Irish priests in Srinagar and later trained in Germany at Mercedes-Benz, was a first rate mechanic and mountaineer who spoke the dialects of the region. The garden smelt of roses. The chant of fishermen sailed across the air and evening clouds, singed with red, dappled the sky.

Then I was in Amarnath. On the way into Ladakh, Nazir and I had joined pilgrims en route to a sacred cave. Every year, at the time of the August moon, thousands of Hindus make the journey to pray to Shiva, the god of death and renewal, and ensure a better reincarnation. He is symbolised by a phallic-shaped, iced stalagmite that rises from a spring in the grotto. This Tantric image of life represents creation through the womb of time. I learnt that Tantric symbolism as well as the doctrine of reincarnation gradually flowed from its Hindu source into the tributary of Buddhism.

Finally I saw the Sadu, immobile, naked, covered in ash and oblivious to the cold. He sat in trance. Such masters of Yoga demonstrate control over their subtle energies. This discipline is adopted by the Buddhists. The Sadu was yet another link in the chain relating Tibetan Lamaism to its Vedic past, when Buddhist philosophers left Kashmir to spread their doctrine in the Himalayan kingdoms.

INTO THE ZANGSKAR VALLEY

Now, at dawn, the ranges of Afghanistan were creased together in colours of silk taffeta; pastel blues shaded into mauve. A short stopover in Kabul, and on to Delhi and Srinagar. Nazir was there, his arms wide in welcome. I felt as if we were already half way to the Amchi's mountain. Packed into his jeep, we honked through the back streets with wooden, high-roofed Turkish-style houses and boothes selling pastries and fly-blown meat. The odour of curry and open gutters hit my nostrils, and my senses awakened in the colour and the activity of the East.

We wound our way out of the city, past the floating vegetable gardens to pass the great mosque alongside the lake, after which we came to the garden with the houseboats. The gates scraped open. Abdul was there to meet us.

That evening, moonlight shone on the lake. Waterbirds ceased to twitter, and only a few ducks gave reassuring quacks in answer to the last call from the mosque. We took a 'shikara', the Kashmiri gondola, and paddled across the water. Nazir lit his narghile; it gurgled as he sucked the thin pipe between our shared confidences.

The air was silk against my skin. Tomorrow came the journey for Ladakh and all softness would be left behind.

Dawn had barely broken, when Abdul, warm as toast in his grey cloak, provided us with chicken and hot bread. We loaded the jeep, and an hour later, with Gulam and Mohamet, our cook and tent boy, we drove off shouting 'We will return'. 'In's Allah!' came the chorused reply. Our search for the living traditions of Tibetan medicine had begun. The road would take us through time and space, through lands of Muslim tribes, and on into the mountain strongholds of Ladakhi Buddhists.

'So!' said Nazir, 'last time you arrived to work, but never sent me any of your pictures.' I apologised. 'But this time it seems to be different,' he went on, 'has something happened to bring you back again?' Although Nazir had frequently regaled me with ribald episodes from his numerous affairs we had rarely discussed personal feelings but now I quickly explained my changed situation and said that I intended to write an article on a Tibetan Amchi. 'Fine! Are you telling me that you'll end up with a book about how you went into the mountains and found God?' he asked. As usual by intent or instinct he had hit on target. Behind the trappings of my profession lay a real quest to find a wider view of the patterns of life. Patterns giving meaning not by mere philosophy but from the intimate revelations of experience. So simple yet so difficult unless I was able to ask the correct questions. I reached out and touched Nazir's arm. '*You* are an extraordinary friend,' I said.

And so we entered the Himalayas, a grander Switzerland. After refreshment at Sonamarg, 'The Golden Fields', so named from the Spring crocus that cover the grass, we drove up onto the plateau. A puncture, and a jammed gear box slowed us down. Gulam and Mohamet went into a huddle with Nazir over the engine. We were saved by the arrival of a lorry, and hitched up with a worn piece of rope, we hurtled behind the load of sheep peering stupidly at us through wooden bars. By hard hooting we made the driver understand that we wished to be brought to Kargil, an outpost in this world, and not the portals of heaven.

A dreary, dreadful dump of a town, Kargil was a halt for army lorries and other transport. Next morning, the mountains came to life as if born that very night to rise and flow around us. 'Going into the Zangskar, are you?' said our inn keeper. 'Well you'll see, we Muslims are richer and more powerful than the Buddhists because we have more children. In a few years there will be a mosque in every Ladakhi village.' He served a reasonable breakfast offering us the privilege of applying local honey to soggy, white bread. The bill showed his unswerving devotion to commerce and to skinning travellers. The price was higher than a kite over Everest.

'You Westerners value worldly success. We value the inner man,' had said an old Lama on my previous visit. It would be naive to think that the Buddhists have no interest in making money. Ladakh, opened to tourism in 1974, was ripe for theft and the illicit sales of temple treasures. Before the Indian government catalogued the valuables in the monasteries, the monks had not the faintest idea of their worth. The unscrupulous made a fast buck in selling faked antique tankas or painted silk icons for a price without compassion. 'They'll get their just desserts, if not in this life then the next!' said my Ladakhi friends without rancour.

With our jeep hopelessly out of order, Nazir booked us on a lorry in a convoy of five vehicles. 'There'll be six of us in the drivers cabin.' he said. 'So count yourself lucky to be small and thin because we'll be having a joy-ride over 240 kilometres. Beautiful scenery, horrid road!'

After another night in a sleazy hotel, we rose at day break. The stars shivered in the dawn, and from the mosque the first call to prayer floated out in arabesques of sound. It struck an atavistic cord. All ugliness vanished in that cry, and for a moment Kargil became a caravanserai for modern nomads. A thunderous overture of revved engines and shouts from the late-comers running out of houses to toss baggage into the lorries, announced our imminent departure. The roar of motors replaced bygone camel bells, but the atmosphere of adventure remained.

Hours later, we halted for breakfast under the snowy peaks of Nun and Kun, two white teeth that bit into the blue bowl of the sky. Were these mountains so young that their bare flanks had not yet grown a cover, or was it rock-bones that roasted in the sun? All rigidity of time became specious in this mineral world unchanged since the mythic age when gods descended to teach man their medicine. We were journeying back into the middle ages towards a terrain at the top of the world, amid peaks and valleys that could have belonged to another planet.

Village mosques soon gave way to small monasteries, their tattered prayer flags waving messages to heaven in the all pervasive presence of Buddhism . . . and dust. Houses of mud over sun-baked brick had flat roofs insulated with twigs. Along a river, fields of barley formed strips of faded green, so brave in their wild setting. In this landscape of essentials, I at last felt able to feel at one with myself. Petty thoughts and recriminations, irritating offspring of the mind, and superficial shadows of a corrosive materialism vanished as I became more and more aware of the vast space about us. There was no room for them here. Challenging even the will to survive, this land offered no easy welcome. Its contrast to the accustomed props of my existence threw me back onto myself. Small wonder that 'Gompa', the Tibetan word for monastery means 'a solitary place'.

Our slow pace gave time for an inner acclimatisation to a culture that had remained intact for centuries. Nature's medicines were everywhere, their abundance a witness to the wealth of traditional cures rooted in vegetable, animal and mineral substances. I watched the sleek marmots sunning themselves by the road. Their livers are eaten to help mend cracked bones. Lizards streaked between rocks; their flesh cures kidney ailments. Hawks wheeled over head; their meat calms nausea. Snake flesh prevents constipation and eye maladies, its skin holds properties for lucodemia and the fat helps in the extraction of bullets. Plants and herbs, the mainstay of Tibetan pharmacology, grew from this hard earth, and mineral waters gushed over blistered rocks. It pleased me that Buddhism had left the fatalism and resignation of India for this land whose people had prospered from their resources and their faith. From these perspectives, my troubles dwindled in importance. A herd of small, mud-encrusted ponies, their manes and tails blowing in the wind, raced over a hill, away from the roar of the convoy. A mythological pedigree claims their birth from the streams tumbling down the summit of the Pensi-la, the pass that was leading us into the Zangskar.

Our lorry broke its axle negotiating a steep bend. 'Damn it!' hissed Nazir, 'Playtime over. On to work. I'll help the men. But I bet Zangskar farmers are saying we deserve all we've got since we didn't ask the gods' permission when we dug out the road and moved the boulders a mile back. They'll say the earth demons have cursed us.' 'The people making this road didn't put in enough effort for our security.' I retorted ironically, but on reflection, I thought that asking permission to disturb the earth's tranquillity was a way of giving homage to a support for life, an element we did not create but can destroy.

By dusk, on the second day, we came to the ramshackle outskirts of Padum, the ancient capital of the Zangskar kingdom. Chortens,

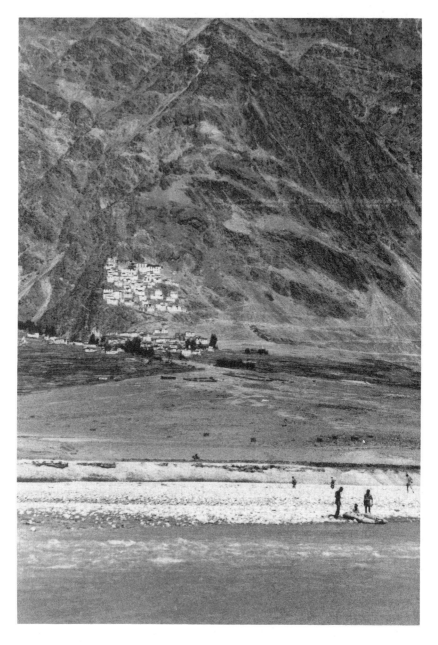

Karsha

harbouring the relics of saintly men, dotted the landscape. The monuments, symbols of Buddhist philosophy, are designed in five sections to bear witness to the five Elements of Creation. The principle of Earth represents the body; Water, its fluids; Fire, its heat; Air, its life and movement; and Space, its area for growth. Each section has a mystic and medical significance.

Throughout Ladakh, the Buddhists felt threatened in their identity and culture by the onslaught of Indian administration and the trading acumen of Islamic society. I, the stranger, with no one to threaten my identity, had come to absorb whatever I could, and had chosen Tibetan medicine as my guide.

We had arrived in a closed society with few contacts beyond the valley. Tractors, and the radios of government officials had done little to change the lives of the people committed to seasonal occupations on the land. They walked or rode into Padum for provisions and news from Kashmiri and Sikh traders. Occasionally, the farmers and herders went off to Kargil or Leh, the capital, otherwise, distant hamlets were united at festivals in a culture that taught reverence for life, and gentleness and hospitality to strangers.

With our bones still aching from the convoy, after a night in Padum, we marched off early, Gulam and Mohamet carrying enormous loads for the six mile walk to the river we had to cross to reach Karsha. The wind, so similar to my own behavior under stress, came up in sudden menace, dust clouding the sky. Half an hour later, as fast as it had arisen, the storm subsided in worn-out puffs, exhausted from hurling its bad temper across a land too vast to care. Small figures, we trekked over the plain hedged in by mountains, their formations frozen into giant ripples. By midday we had reached the river, a beige and silver barrier between us and our destination. The crossing was a nightmare. A race against time as the ferrymen paddled us over the strong current in a rapidly deflating dinghy.

On the other side, we relaxed on stones resembling a thousand dinosaurs eggs. When dry and rested, we made camp nearby. I looked up at the village; no mirage, it sat embedded in the side of a thundering mountain. Only the Amchi remained to pass from my imagination into reality, and on the arrival of an inquisitive shepherd, Nazir asked him for directions to the Amchi's home. He pointed to a cluster of white farm houses in a clump of trees a mile from our camp. An array of expectations came to mind. My heart beat faster. I wondered what manner of man would appear. Would he welcome us or were we mad to expect acceptance from a stranger? Perhaps he would consider us impolite to presume that he had the time and the inclination to instruct us? Soon we would know.

ONE

•

The meeting with Sonam, the Amchi—He initiates us into the mysteries of Tibetan medicine, its texts and how he was trained as a doctor

OUR MEETING WITH SONAM, THE AMCHI

Sonam, the Amchi, walked out of his little white house and paused by the gate waiting for us to approach him. His burgundy robe was corded at the waist, yak skin boots covered his legs and on his head perched a velvet stove-pipe hat with sides turned up like the wings of a pagoda. No outward insignia marked his profession. He looked at us with eyes narrowed against the sunlight, his face serene yet inquisitive as he slowly fingered a rosary of wooden beads. His hands were beautiful.

Nazir introduced me as a friend of the TV producer who had filmed him a few months ago. After our hard journey he hoped that the Amchi might give us the honour of being with him for a short time to learn something of his medicine. The Amchi raised his head slightly and his eyes passed slowly from Nazir to myself. When a small girl came to peer at us from behind his robe, without removing his gaze his hand went down to stroke her head. Silent and still, he took his time before giving an answer. With a brief nod and a disarming smile, he beckoned us into the house. We mounted the steps accompanied by more children and entered a small, neat room scented by dried herbs hanging from the rafters. A bed covered with sheepskin, two chairs, a rug and boxes by the window left just enough room for a table. His clothes hung from a peg and magazine pictures of the Dalai Lama were the only decoration.

When we had settled down on the floor near the window, Sonam

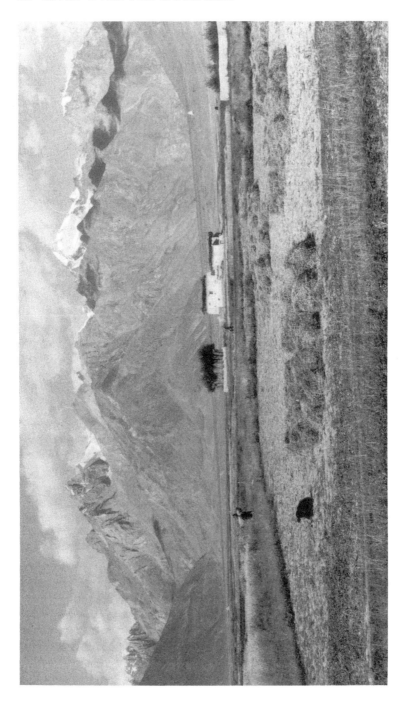

Sonam's house with the barley field

asked Nazir if I had brought the photos promised by John Roberts. Knowing nothing about them, I said no, and was embarrassed by Sonam's transparent disappointment. 'A promise is something sacred in Ladakh,' Nazir whispered to me, 'Your friend should have been more considerate.'

After a few minutes of discussion between the two men, Nazir turned towards me, his face split in an enormous grin: 'The Amchi has agreed to take us with him tomorrow morning on his rounds in the villages.' I thanked him profusely, and wondered to what extent curiosity had played a part in his decision. Except for John and the TV team, Sonam's contact with Europeans in this remote valley was limited to trekkers. I had seldom come across anyone whose curiosity about foreigners extended further than asking them their names and number of children. I was relieved to have been spared these details.

A good looking woman wearing a dark robe sashed with pink and a scarf over her plaits, came in with tea and biscuits. She was the Amchi's sister. 'Dolka has cared for the house since my wife's death,' explained Sonam, 'my daughter is married to a farmer, my eldest son is a school teacher and my other son is preparing to enter the monastery.' A young boy dressed in a robe, with a woollen cap on his head, rushed through the door and bowed his way to sit at the Amchi's feet. He was introduced as Thelmy, the Amchi's fourteen year-old nephew and apprentice. 'He goes to school in summer, and I teach him from our sacred texts in winter when we are snowed in. Like all boys, he is happiest outside the classroom and in the holidays he visits the patients with me.'

THE MYSTERIES OF TIBETAN MEDICINE

Traditionally, a disciple follows his master for five to seven years in a relationship requiring patience and devotion with no material rewards. Basic knowledge is learnt by heart, and by going with the master into the mountains, the aspiring Amchi is progressively initiated into herbal lore. Tibetan doctors are both pharmacologists and dieticians. Unlike their Western counterparts, they use no instruments for diagnosis.

'We train our senses over a period of ten years,' explained Sonam, replenishing his tea. He spoke softly, but when the children began squabbling, he rose, clapped his hands and ordered them from the room. Beneath his gentleness lay the authority of a patriarch. Beyond his simplicity I sensed no place for familiarity. 'Our fingers become like seeing ears,' he continued, pausing to watch our reaction, 'we take the body's pulses, and from their beat we diagnose illness. Each internal organ has its own pulse felt by holding the patient's wrists. I know you do not understand how this is done. But, no matter, we will discuss it all later.' The Amchi looked at me. 'I have told you this first because it was the aspect of our medicine that most fascinated your friend John Roberts.'

Sonam pointed to a brocade wrapped package on the shelf above his bed, and Thelmy, unprompted, leapt up and brought it over. Uncovered, it revealed four sets of long and narrow block-printed pages held between carved, wooden covers. 'These are the sacred teachings of the Buddha transmitted by a long line of sages. We have gathered them into four great books of medicine we call the Four Tantras.[1] They should all be learnt by heart. In Tibetan, Tantra, in its medical context, means 'that which enlarges knowledge'. Our four books are here to protect the body, and our eight branches of medicine deal with all the body's functions, the diseases of children and women, and illness caused by evil spirits, wounds, accidents and poisons.' He smiled, 'We also have a section on rejuvenation and fertility for people of both sexes. Use these teachings well and they will flower in health and longevity. Use them wisely and they will ripen into the fruits of spiritual insight, prosperity and happiness.'

The first book, or 'Root Tantra' is supposedly only for people of high intelligence. This idea may be a relic of the Vedic caste system. The top caste are the hereditary Brahmins, who to this day think they have the right to exclusive knowledge. Sonam, however, was not here to judge our intelligence, but to give us insight into the Buddha's medical teachings. He added that the student who memorises the first book becomes a 'small doctor', unless its deeper significance is understood. This 'Root Tantra' contains the essence of all the oral instruction developed in the second volume, enlarged in the third, and put into ready reference for immediate consultation in the fourth.[2] Students may study for up to nine years. There is no concept of specialisation. After graduation, a doctor remains in contact with his master for the rest of his life.

Sonam had not studied as an apprentice to a village Amchi, usually an hereditary profession, but with the Abbot of the

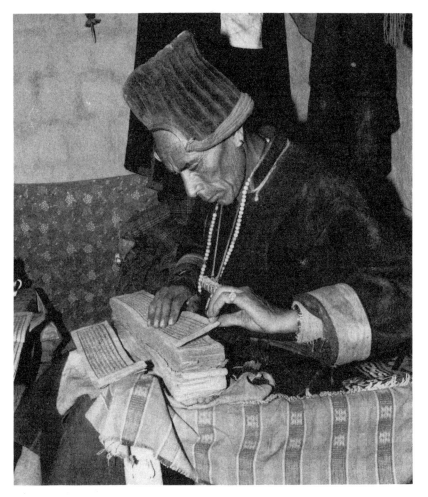

Sonam with texts

monastery. After seven years he had mastered theory in anatomy, embryology, physiology, pathology, therapies and medicines. When he finally graduated he was given the title of Amchi – a Mongolian word meaning doctor – and enjoyed a great celebration in Karsha. Invested with approval of both the Abbot and the village elders, he was introduced into the community as their new doctor.

'Did you take an oath?' I asked.

'Oh yes! It is a most important moment. We say, I swear to fight all forms of suffering with perseverance and compassion and perpetual vigour. Even now after twelve years I return as often as possible to the monastery and continue to learn more from commentaries and philosophical works.'

Sonam adjusted his hat and rose in silence and we went out into the fading light. At the gate, he said, if time permitted, he would come and visit our camp in the evening after he had prepared his medicines and found horses for tomorrow's trip.

EFFECTS BECOME CAUSES

The walk back took us past fields of barley ready for harvest. We were met in camp by a gaggle of children and two women loaded with firewood gathered from the bushes on the stony hills below Karsha, which was perched in orange against a purple mountain. No sooner had I crawled into my tent than the flaps were lifted and impish little faces peered in to observe my every move. Joined by the women, the youngsters drew aside to let their elders look at my underclothes and toilet articles. When I placed a bottle of scent under their noses, they grimaced. I cut the nails of one girl, and in thanks she and her playmates gave a boisterous rendition of 'Frere Jacques' learnt from French trekkers, but my attempts to organise them in a round threw the choir into chaos and shrieks of laughter.

At Gulam's arrival with a basin of hot water, my audience vanished and their chatter faded into the distance. Clean and warmly dressed, I joined the men in the mess tent. To ward off the creeping chill, I helped fill and light the primus stoves and sort out our provisions until our activity stopped on the intrusion of a cold draught. Looking up we saw the Amchi, silent as a phantom, standing in the entrance. Nazir, in welcome, led him to sit on a tin trunk moved next to the lamp. Given a cup of coffee, Sonam opened the conversation by asking where my husband was. 'Tell him my husband has bolted with another woman,' I said. At Nazir's short and sharp reply, the Amchi roared with laughter. Between guffaws, the good doctor's answer made my gallant interpreter snigger and hesitate before translating. 'He said the woman must have a very fine fire and your husband enjoys being a moth that gets burnt.' 'Do you dislike that lady?' asked the Amchi. For once I was speechless. This man, who appeared so artless in his simplicity and enjoyment of life showed astonishing powers of observation. 'Do not be trapped in ignorance and its mental poisons,' he said, 'you should turn away from aversion for the lady and follow the path of compassion.'

'He hasn't wasted any time in asking about my private life,' I said aside to Nazir, 'how would he like it if I asked him why his wife died?' Nazir shifted his feet and gently replied, 'he isn't delving into your private affairs, he's just come out with a direct question. He's a doctor used to talking openly with people, and your reply gave him a chance to introduce his philosophy. In your case, you are not a doctor, your question is not polite. Perhaps his wife died from an illness he was unable to cure, so let's forget the subject.'

Had anyone proferred the Amchi's advice in my own culture, I would have disregarded it as self-conscious charity delivered in a world where all is fair in love and war – providing one is on the winning side. In the distant setting of a tent in Ladakh, Sonam's words, although gall in my throat, were, nonetheless, more acceptable. Life with my husband, a diplomat, had taken us through the capitals of Europe to Vienna where, homesick for the warmth and fun of Rome, I retreated into nostalgia and watched rooks croak on naked trees under snow tumbling from leaden skies. My humour grew darker by the day on the discovery that my man was beguiled by another woman. We left Vienna, but no-one was spared from the misery. Two homes with children were broken. How could I review the loss of home and husband as the workings of fate and take the antidote of compassion to purge the mind of bitterness. So many times I had tried to pierce through that curtain of mystery to see if I could catch a glimpse of some anterior action which might have shed light on what happened; a near pointless endeavour since all activity has its effect and effects themselves become causes.

REINCARNATION

'Man is offered knowledge and instruction,' the Amchi continued, 'so that he can be in harmony with himself and his surroundings. When actions deviate from the Buddha's teachings, sooner or later the results take the form of illness. Until ignorance is eliminated, the body can never be completely healthy. If I succumb to anger, my behaviour and actions will be negative and bring about an imbalance in my constitution. While we prepare pain and pleasure to be experienced now and in a future incarnation, some of the unhappy and unfortunate occurrences in this life result from what we did in past existences'.

The concept of reincarnation which he referred to was in no way strange to me. Often in my childhood I had had visions of myself in strange places and wearing clothes of a past era. These visions could be unleashed by a painting, a story, a place. They triggered a flow of images as if I watched a film, coloured and in three dimensions. Nothing could prove they had any more reality than a dream, yet the scenes were real for me, and I kept silent to avoid derision. Then, in my early teens, recovering from pneumonia, I was tutored by our farm manager's wife. A qualified biologist, widely read, who introduced me to reincarnation. It all made sense.

'If this is so,' I remarked to Sonam, 'what a shame that most of us can't recall our mistakes. I am sure we go on perpetuating the same stupidities because we have forgotten the consequences.'

Sonam looked at me with merriment. 'Just as well! If you remember, good. If not, it doesn't matter. It means you are not yet ready for it, and anyway, you must deal with life in the present, using what you know. If you meet a deformed beggar, would you dismiss his misery as the price paid for his bad Karma and refuse him your compassion, or a rupee? You speak of repeated mistakes, well, it is true, and the same situation will come about again and again unless you have learnt your lesson. Unpleasant or pleasant, Karma is not simple. It stems from innumerable, interdependent factors.

'Are you saying if I don't master my reactions and forgive that the same problem and the same people will face me in the next incarnation?'

'Possibly. It depends on all kinds of internal and external conditions, and the force of your emotions. We have to go on learning from the experiences of life after life until understanding becomes distilled in our consciousness. There are people who are born "knowing", even if they don't remember. Others have recall but don't always recognise the implications. A few remember and understand and have chosen rebirth to help others. In the end, you cannot teach anyone anything that they don't know already!'

'All this food for thought has not filled my stomach. I'm rave-nous,' said Nazir. He sniffed the meal and bent towards the Amchi, asking him to dine with us. Sonam declined. He had eaten at home. The lamplight, heightened by candles, transformed his head and robe into a Georges de la Tour painting. Captivated by the blurred outlines, almost liquid in the way they shifted through shades of colour, I imagined the change of tones transposed into music. Disinclined to talk, I hoped Nazir would engage our guest in conversation, while I, safe in the shadows, could relax into silence. But Sonam was clearly ready for more dialogue. Ignorance, he had mentioned, spawned mental poisons, which, if not flushed from the mind, flourish abundantly.

With my mind a complete blank quite incapable of framing any kind of perceptive question, I felt disoriented, and unable to dir-ectly connect our different ways of thinking, I clumsily blurted out, 'Nazir, ask him about mental poisons, will you?' As the words left my mouth, I knew that no matter what Sonam said, his tacit comprehension of all things familiar to him since childhood which had no place in my culture, could only be appreciated on my part intellectually. From his earliest instruction, the measure of his thought and action was founded on reincarnation caused by Ignor-ance. The repercussion of this spiritual blindness accompanied by the mental poisons could hardly be restricted to a single existence since a procession of lives spanned a time beyond our consider-ations. Sonam would have been perplexed by our psychology which takes no longer view of man's aberrations than that they might begin from the foetus' experience in the womb. Then marked by our inherited traits, education and life's traumas, we bear the consequences which evaporate at death. I felt like a squirrel with a horde of nuts. I knew their shapes but their taste escaped me.

Before answering, Sonam introduced us to the basic constituents of our being. The body is an organism that mirrors the activity of the universe: a microcosm born from the five Cosmic Elements of the macrocosm. Earth, Fire, Water, Air and Aether (Space). These five are channelled into three forces known as the 'Nopas'. The Wind Nopa is associated with life and consciousness. Its qua-lity is neutral; The Bile Nopa is associated with the body's heat and blood; its quality is cool. Wind is not the air we breathe, nor Bile and Phlegm the body's actual secretions. Like the Cosmic Elements, they are principles recognised by their qualities and functions.

THE THREE NOPAS

'In Tibetan,' explained the Amchi, 'the word ''Nopa'' means ''that which harms'' which shows why we regard our body's behaviour as being far from perfect. The Nopas are influenced by diet, behaviour, the seasons and the positions of the stars and the planets. A state of mind also disrupts a Nopa's disposition. Now, to answer your question: The Wind Nopa is upset by Desire, the Bile Nopa by Anger, the Phlegm Nopa by Delusion, or if you like, Confusion.'

Sonam raised his hand to his chest, 'The principle of the Wind Nopa is the life-giving breath of the Universe projected into our bodies'. His hand moved to his forehead. 'The Wind Nopa clarifies the senses and the mind, passes downwards to help the digestion. Its mental poison is Desire, seated in the genitals. The Bile Nopa keeps the internal organs in touch with each other, directs the body's heat, and among other things, colours the hair. Its poison is Anger seated in the heart. The Phlegm Nopa keeps the joints supple and helps you sleep. If it is disturbed in conjunction with the Wind Nopa, it causes gastric problems. Its poison is Delusion seated in the brain. You surely have had sleepless nights when your mind is agitated.'

I no longer saw my body as a discreet entity. According to Sonam, the substantial and the ephemeral both partook of the same reality. His theories contained a fluidity of concepts that floated in a perpetual interchange of subtle energies. Man, by fact of his constitution, was woven from and into the fabric of the Cosmos, and biological function was an expression of metaphysical powers acting through the human organism. The trouble with Western thought is that it is too compartmentalised, I reflected. Friends group together by profession. The young housewife with children bemoans her enclosure and wants to break out into other categories of life. The overworked long for vacations. The old, trundled out of society, fade into obscurity. The lonely remain isolated in front of their TV sets. I, one of those lucky people who worked at home at the kitchen table, was used to jumping from sorting photos to cooking or to talking with my daughter and friends in for supper. Privileged and unfettered, I travelled extensively. My life was supple, my balance precarious. Suppleness and balance, the secret of a dancer's success and a rewarding life, were the same qualities that Sonam sought to maintain in the the bodies and minds of those he attended. Relating mental states to illness, he relied on the

'Dharma', the Buddha's teachings on thought and behaviour as a guide for coping with human weakness.

'Everything we do in stupidity or wisdom has its consequences. When we are moral and guided by devotion, generosity and a purity of firm intention, we think correctly. Our actions and words are not contradictory, nor do they harm anyone, and . . . our three bodies are in harmony,' he said.

'Three bodies?' I exclaimed.

'We are composed of three distinct but inseparable bodies; mental, subtle and physical,' explained Sonam. 'Ignorance perturbs thought and thought acts on the invisible energy body that circulates within us the universal forces directing life and matter. The subtle works on the material, so if the subtle body is upset it affects the physical state. We deal with this interacting triad of mind, energy and matter in the three aspects of our medicine. I have touched on the mental and moral factors. The subtle body is invigorated and purified by meditation, prayer and the methods of breathing taught in Tantric Medicine, while we use medicines, therapies, diet and, in rare cases, surgery for the outward manifestations of illness.'

Still intrigued by the Nopas, I asked if they affected our physical characteristics. 'Yes,' he answered. 'Our texts say that a Phlegm natured person has a cool, fat body, a large tall frame and a pale complexion. His carriage is upright and he can withstand hunger, thirst and mental stress. He lives long and sleeps well. Often he reacts slowly and bears a grudge. He is also kind with good intentions. His sign is the chief buffalo in the herd, the lion or the mythical Garuda bird.

'People with a predominant Wind Nopa are often bent in posture, dark, talkative and dislike cold wind. Riches escape them. Their life can be short. They love music and laughter. Their emblem is the vulture, raven or fox.

'The Bile Nopa makes people fierce and full of pride. They sweat easily and have a strong odour; their stature is medium. Their life span and wealth are average. Their animal is the tiger or the monkey.'

The Nopas seemed to be a cosmic genetic blue-print which impressed on their bearers distinct physical and psychological traits. In looking at the Amchi I wondered which Nopa ruled his constitution. Our short acquaintance made it difficult to say. His medium height and thin, fine-boned physique clearly ruled out Phlegm, but he was kind and benevolent. Bile? No. There was none of the tiger or monkey in him, nor obvious pride, and his body smelt of dust and herbs. That left Wind, and although his posture was straight and his skin light where unbronzed by the sun, there was something of the fox's and raven's alertness in his face and bearing. He also talked and laughed with ease.

'Honoured Amchi, is your predominant Nopa, Wind?' I asked.

'It is,' he answered. 'but few of us conform to the simple definitions I have given. There are numerous ramifications and we generally are a mixture with a slight tendency for one Nopa to rule over the others'.

The Nopas flow through our body in three invisible channels. A further network of up to 100 000 passages (the Indian 'Nadi') fans out across our organism. It transmits supra energy into the blood, the bodily fluids and the air that sustains life. Its subtle patterns have been captured on paper by Kirlian photography, and apart from recording the flow emitted from fingertips and toes, this technique shows the varying intensity of emanations according to an individual's general state. Impending sickness is detected before the physical symptoms appear. The same effects have been noted in plants and animals.

The Tibetans had taken the concept of these mystic energies from the Hindus, who, in the second millenia before Christ, called the life force 'Prana'. They charted and categorised its course within the flesh directing its power by breath control. When I told the Amchi about Kirlian photography, he admitted knowing very little about western medicine other than it relied a lot on machines.

'What you have told me is not surprising. I have been to the hospital in Leh. One of my friends is a doctor there, a Tibetan trained in Srinagar. He showed me the X-ray machines and many of your other "supports" for diagnosis and, I must say, exquisite instruments for surgery. We believe that to cut into the body results in too much shock, besides, our methods are crude next to yours. Operations were virtually abandoned after a heart operation on the king's mother in the ninth century. But, very occasionally I remove cataracts although I prefer to take my patients to Leh. It is better. And,' he laughed, 'I like the journey. The change is good. I see old friends, we talk and I hear news. The Indian government has opened a school for Amchis there, not very good. Too many young people today want to learn everything fast. When I was twenty years-old, the village elders decided I should present myself to the monks because they thought I was bit more clever than most.' He rubbed his chin and chuckled as if he had commented on someone other than himself. 'I would have gone to Lhasa had the political climate been better, but it was wiser to stay in the Zangskar. The frontiers were already hard to cross.' 'Do you regret not having gone to Tibet?' I asked. 'Of course I do. I wanted to see the Potala Palace, and the two medical colleges. The most famous was Chakpuri built under the fifth Dalai Lama near four hundred years ago. It was the beginning of a public health service in Tibet and the first medical college outside the monasteries. The Chinese destroyed it in 1959. They left the second institute of Mendze Khan, founded by the thirteenth Dalai Lama early in this century. I also hear that Mendze Khan, the House of Astronomy and Medicine, has been improved by the Communists, probably because they respect our medicine. It has roots in common with their own traditions. In the old days, their texts on herbs and pulses added information to ours, and in return, our pharmacology interested them. I understand they removed some of the faculties to the new hospital in Lhasa. Unfortunately, the Chinese do not permit research on the relationship between mind and body, which for us, is indispensable, as I have tried to explain.'

Tibetan medicine, isolated for four centuries, had only come into contact with western systems after the Chinese invasion in 1951, and later, in the mass exodus of 1955. 'How do you get your news?' I asked.

'At least twice a year in the Zangskar, Amchis from all over Ladakh and as far away as Nepal, gather here to exchange herbs. Our valleys are noted for their medicinal plants. We exchange news and discuss cures and barter ingredients. One Amchi told me that the Chinese have begun cultivating medicinal plants on a high altitude farm near Lhasa. They have made a book of coloured photographs.' Sonam fingered his rosary. He looked pensive. 'My aged uncle was trained at Mendze Khan. He now lives in the Tibetan community at Daramsala where His Holiness, our Dalai Lama, started a hospital in 1961. Today, if young men and women want to learn medicine but can't go there, they become apprentices to an Amchi or study in the monasteries of Ladakh, Nepal or Bhutan. In my uncle's time, during the 1930s, Mendze Khan accommodated 150 students.'

'Wasn't it an institute for astrology?' asked Nazir passing the Amchi another cup of tea.

'Astrology has its place in our medicine. Mendze Khan was the first college to produce official calendars. We have recorded twenty-eight constellations, remember, I told you the Nopas are affected by the seasonal position of planets and stars. They transmit the cosmic powers of creation and destruction, or, as I like to say, the influences of transformation. The sages had good reason to teach astrology with medicine. A birth chart helps tell us what can be done to improve a child's constitution. Certain medicines given just after birth, can help mental and physical development; my uncle even spoke of letters representing sounds that when placed under an infant's tongue, would invoked the vibrations of that lettersound and increase the intellect. More important, astrologers foretold remarkable events that touched the nation. When they knew extraordinary incarnations were about to take place, the children were located and educated for top administrative posts. A birth chart can equally give warning of an evil incarnation. We believe that after the reign of the thirteenth Dalai Lama, astrology has not been well used in Tibet.'

Students, in his uncle's day, he told us, rose at 3 am to say prayers and recite astronomical texts until 6 am. After breakfast came grammar, medicine, writing and poetry. After lunch, they observed patients brought to the college, and had classes in anatomy, mathematics, geometry and the history of medicine. Training lasted never less than six years with annual written and oral examinations. Those who failed were given another chance. Seasonal excursions took students into the mountains to collect herbs, and on days of special festivals, they danced in honour of the Buddha of Medicine.

'It makes me exhausted just thinking of what those people had to learn each day. I doubt if any of them had more than six hours sleep a night.' said Nazir, stifling a yawn.

It was late. Sonam made a slight bow and raised his hand as if in blessing before he strode out into the night, his figure erect against the wind.

'What a strange fellow!' Nazir continued, 'rather different from other Amchis I have come across in Ladakh. They are rough country herbalists and not very well trained. Exceptions like Sonam prove the rule. Under his simple ways, I think he hides a very strong character.'

'And, a generous nature,' I added. 'Did you noticed the gap between his front teeth? They say it's a sign of great generosity.'

The concept of generosity, emphasised the fact that I had left a world obsessed by quantity to enter a culture where quality suffused thought, as well as designating the attributes of life.

NOTES

[1] *The Tantras.* Tantra in the conversational sense means the employment of ritual to gain the aid of powers personified by demons or gods. Communication takes place through the use of images, gestures and prayers of invocation. Tantric Buddhism is a magico-mystical discipline applied either in sorcery or to obtain enlightenment. Sonam's tabulation of the different aspects of life dealt with in Tibetan medicine included illness caused by evil spirits. In this sense one could apply the classic meaning of Tantra

[2] The Four Tantras, or in Tibetan, the *Rgyud-bzhi,* were written in four-lined stanzas of nine syllables and put into their present form under the guidance of the Regent of the fifth Dalai Lama towards the end of the seventeenth century. Current medical practices were added to earlier translations from the Indian and Chinese texts. To make them more easily understood, the texts were rewritten as a dialogue between two sages in mythical times. The books transmit the teaching of the Buddha in his penultimate incarnation.

TWO

———————•———————

*We leave on horseback with the Amchi on his
rounds to the villages—He explains the theory
of the Elements—He gives his version of the
history of his medicine, his views on cancer
and administers a therapeutic bath—Healing
is welded to religion*

The Amchi rode into our camp at dawn. He arrived on a white
stallion followed by his nephew Thelmy leading a third horse.
Once the provisions had been strapped over our wooden saddles,
he and Thelmy went off at a fast trot, the boy astride the rump
of his uncle's stallion. They broke into a canter across a landscape
of such splendour that I reined in to take a photo. At the same
moment, my bedding which was balanced on the saddle slid to
the ground. No matter, I didn't need a camera to remember these
mountains, mauve and tipped with snow, or this valley with its
artery of silver water carrying life to a land of stones traversed
by the sorcerer and his apprentice.

Laden with bags and camera equipment, Nazir, boots touching
the ground, sat astride a minute pony. His floppy hat added the
final touch to a picture of utter dejection as his mare lifted her
tail for a string of pathetic farts that punctuated her dreary progress
in a vista no longer grand, but desolate. Somehow this scene gave
the right tone to our expedition. On no account were we to take
ourselves seriously; only the quest mattered. Nazir was the first
to agree.

The wind whipped our faces and I was exhilarated in my contact
with the rawness of the air, the dry heat and the view of distant
water. Sonam had dismounted and waited crouched down next

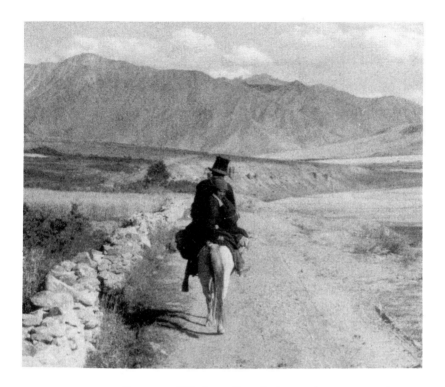

Sonam and Thelmy off on their rounds

to a white-washed, five-tiered chorten of considerable size. Chortens date back to the eighth century when they were first constructed as beacons to the Buddha's presence. In time, they became shrines for the relics of holy men, and built on barren heights along trails through passes, or lined up along farmlands and in villages, they usually mark the path to a monastery.

THE COSMIC ELEMENTS

'Chortens are emblems of the law,' said Sonam. 'They represent the five constituents of the universe and man standing between the upper worlds and earth. Man mediates between the spiritual and earthly forces. His body contains the powers of Earth, Water, Fire, Air and Space. Our medicine tries to keep them in harmony.'

ELEMENT	CHAKRA	PRINCIPLE	SENSE	COLOUR	ZONE
SPACE	CROWN	CHANGE	HEARING	WHITE	SUPERIOR
AIR	THROAT	MOVE-MENT	TOUCH	GREEN	INTERMEDIARY
FIRE	HEART	HEAT	SIGHT	RED	
WATER	SOLAR PLEXUS	FLUIDITY	TASTE	BLUE	
EARTH	RECTO GENITAL	STABILITY	SMELL	YELLOW	INFERIOR

Chortens as emblems of the law

'Are these elements you talk about those we know in everyday life?' questioned Nazir.

'No. The soil and rivers, the fire under the pots and the air and space around you are only their earthly aspects. They must not be confused with their parents, the Cosmic Elements of Creation. Man shares these cosmic constituents with the land he inhabits. In one sense, we are separated from the Elements because our consciousness is human, but we are never untouched by their effects. Our whole being has been formed from their essence.'

Bones, flesh and muscle and our sense of smell come from the Earth Element, the supportive agent. Earth solidifies, Water lubricates, Fire heats, Air brings movement and Space is the Element that allows growth.

The Water Element carries the qualities of weight, suppleness, coolness and holds matter together in all manner of forms. Water is responsible for the formation of body liquids and engenders our sense of taste. Fire, the maturing agent, is linked to the sun that fosters growth. It directs the body's temperature, influences pigmentation and gives birth to our sense of sight. Air is responsible for the breathing process fundamental to life. Its subtle energy *is* life. Intimately associated with our skin, Air brings forth our sense of touch. Space, the Element in which every animate and inanimate form, every type of manifestation comes into being, exists, grows, changes, dies, and reappears again in a different state, also constitutes the body's cavities and gives rise to the sense of sound. Simplicity may well guard great wisdom, I thought, but this theory, though true to itself, still left me in a quandary.

'Our theory is not complicated,' said Sonam, 'the five Elements reflect themselves in the body. They give birth to the senses and transport their qualities through their messengers we call the "Nopas." At certain junctions of the "Nopas" are the energy centres of "Khor-lo" that the Indians call Chakras. In the Chorten, each of its five sections represents one of the Elements, the sense organ related to it and five of the seven "Khor-lo" '.

The Amchi pointed to the cubic base representing Earth, the body, stability, continuity and vitality. The round shape immediately above, symbolises Water with the fluidity that both carries life and dissolves it. The middle, conical section represents Fire that gives heat and the spark of life. It corresponds to man's position touched by the holy and the profane. The fourth part, an inverted bowl represents Air associated with life, movement and vibration. At the very top, a crescent moon holding the orb of the sun, symbolises the fifth Element, Space (or Aether), the state of transformation, also known as the 'Quintessence of the Sages'. When man is enlightened, his chakras open and all becomes one.

'The Chorten,' said Sonam, 'holds our philosophy as well the bones of saints. Its sections remind us that we are born from the Elements and that the body is merely an envelope for the incarnating being. Existence is like a dream in which we encounter friends and those we dislike. We give ourselves difficulties, avoiding some situations and grabbing at others. They are all phantoms. The body is our dream structured as channels for the cosmic winds of the five Elements. In the most ancient sources, these are but one. When consciousness develops through the senses, our feelings put us in touch with our surroundings, and in the path of evolution we experience pain and happiness, always ephemeral, leading to no final solution until our delusions are forgotten. Individuality is our personal dream. If we can live in harmony and contentment in this dream, so much the better; if we can avoid hurting others, better still.'

A human being is an energy system seeking to gain and retain its equilibrium in many mysterious ways. Our desires cause problems if not kept in order. Man has to cope with forces within himself, within others and in nature. Regardless of our culture, these three factors are parameters of our reality. Whereas Westerners value a sense of self-consciousness, Buddhists think of themselves as vessels for the expression of cosmic order. The culmination of their being is to become one with this order. The five Elements, or principles, act as the underlying dynamics for all material manifestation.

Thelmy leaned over and touched Nazir's sleeve. 'The Buddha's wisdom is here to save us all, even the animals,' he said in his husky voice. Sonam moved to pat the boy's head, a profoundly intimate gesture since it is the seat of the crown chakra, not to be idly touched by strangers. Sonam motioned us to remount. Held up with notes, Nazir and I let them go on ahead.

The breeze blew pleasantly, and he kicked the little mare to keep pace with my more spirited pony. Discussing the ethereal channels that transmit the forces of the Elements, I mentioned that the Yogis – such strange alchemists of the spirit – around 1500 BC, had chartered the supernatural currents of the mystic body within the flesh in an epoch that heralded the concept of reincarnation. 1000 years later, in the seventh century AD, when Buddhism was officially accepted in Tibet, medicine travelled hand in hand with the

Buddhist creed, and its Ayurvedic bones were fleshed with the Tibetans' innovative adaptations and added methods of diagnosis.

Our path snaked through rough hills into a gentle terrain. Around a bend we caught up with the Amchi and Thelmy overcome with laughter. Looking down onto the grasslands, we beheld a singularly obstinate yak and a farmer locked in combat by a cord attached to the beast's nose. Oblivious of the narrow crossing a few yards away, they pulled against each other across an expanse of water. The yak stood inert. The farmer yelled. The tug of war continued for a good minute. Then, with the unexpected attack of a sumo wrestler, the yak plunged into action with a fearful jerk that yanked his enraged master into the stream. The man rose with a curse, and waving his arms, chased after his adversary charging off, tail up, head down, into the wild blue yonder.

Highly amused, Sonam knocked his forehead with his fist, saying, 'Ignorance has many faces but the same head. Those animals have a nasty character, and can rip open a man's belly in a second. Accidents are quite common with the farmers, but if the entrails are not pierced, we can wash them with hot milk and water, put them back in place and sew up the wound with a covering of musk. I have a colleague who once repaired a farmer's head fractured by a kick from his yak. He knew he had to operate fast. My friend removed the smashed piece and replaced it with a well-boiled and polished bone taken from a sheep's skull. The patient is still in the best of health and does not bleat!'

A VISIT TO A SOLDIER

We rode out of the pass onto the plain, and by dusk reached a hamlet. Sonam asked us to wait outside one of the houses as he wanted to explain our presence to his patient, a soldier home on leave. 'The Indian Army has made him very suspicious of foreigners, he thinks you are all spies, so I will put his mind at rest or any treatment will be useless. His stomach complaint comes from eating too much sugar since he was a child. Diet is an essential part of our medicine, and we say a good digestion is the basis of good health. It's a pity he did not come to me earlier because now his cure will take up to at least eight months.' Sonam swung off the stallion followed by Thelmy carrying bedding and the leather medicine pouch that is the badge of an Amchi.

Excited cries of 'Julay' greeted him and we waited quietly until

Sonam came out with the soldier. Thin and obviously ill at ease, his welcome was nevertheless warm and he escorted us into a small, mud-walled room newly built on the side of the house. His grandmother brought in rush matting, clean and sweet smelling, to lay on the dirt floor. The Amchi returned with a thermos of tea and a tin of powdered milk. 'Refresh yourselves and then, if you like, you can come and meet us in the kitchen.' With a slight bow, he withdrew from the doorway.

From the noise and laughter in the kitchen, Sonam's welcome marked his importance as a doctor and friend deeply acquainted with their lives and circumstances. Tibetans are renowned for their pertinent and impertinent comments on human affairs, and by the sound of it, this family had much to recount. We hardly heard Sonam's voice apart from an occasional chuckle. He had come to receive information and not to join in the gossip.

An hour went by before we entered the kitchen, a low, dark room virtually unfurnished with six people sitting by the stove. Sonam was examining the black patches on the face of a young woman; pellagra, caused by malnutrition. He handed her a paste made from fresh butter mixed with the ash of horses hooves. An alternative remedy was sesame oil, milk, tumeric and crushed seeds of black and white cummin. Her diet, he said, would be difficult to afford. She was poor. He would do his best.

Our talk was broken by squeals coming from the front entrance. A small girl, her face streaked with grimy tears, came running to the Amchi. She held out her hand, bitten, she sobbed, by a dog. He picked her up and went outside. 'He has gone to find the dog and make it lick her wound,' explained our host. 'He will then put some ointment on it. We are quite accustomed to this kind of accident.'

Thelmy ran to the Amchi's medicine bag for the ointment kept in an old Nivea tin. He opened it in readiness. On Sonam's return, the child in his arms, he rubbed the paste on the bite, telling us that it was based on bitumen and several herbs, and had been in use for centuries.

'The Persians introduced it into our medicine when they first came to the court of one of our most famous kings almost 1400 years ago,' he said, scraping a portion into a saucer, enough for the next five days. The mother bound her daughter's hand with an old cloth, washed, on Sonam's insistence, in boiling water. Why, we asked, had he made the dog lick the wound? 'We have no explanation in the texts, It is a local custom,' he answered.

Boils, broken bones, infected throats, mumps, measles, lung infections, liver complaints and water retention, arthritis and eye infections were the common complaints he dealt with, but he admitted defeat in what he termed 'degenerative diseases of the bone'.

Whenever he spoke, no one moved. I knew our interest exalted him in their esteem although I never sensed any change in Sonam's attitude. He kept his simple demeanour; no airs of self-importance. I was learning more from his behaviour than from anything that he had said. His manner revealed a man who knew his subject well and had faith in what he practised.

I asked Sonam if he was aware of the West's concern with cancer. 'I understand you have your cures, but in Tibet we recognise that cancer originates in karma. Man is more than his tangible body. He is composed of energy, mind and matter, and when they are not in harmony, confusion enters the consciousness. Unless you can cope with the confusion, you will find more and more terrible diseases appearing to take the place of the one you think you have eliminated. The power of destructive thoughts causes karmic diseases. Among these are cancer, leprosy, and other degenerative diseases, as yet unknown, which will arrive and be caught individually or in epidemics.'

The family nodded in agreement, having followed the conversation intently. Further discussion was interrupted by the grandmother. She asked for help with the sulphur water, transported from the mountains early that morning. The kerosene tins now had to be lifted onto the stove in preparation for the soldier's medicinal bath. As it would take two hours to heat, Sonam suggested we return to our room. He joined us shortly, and installed himself against the wall, his back propped up with a blanket and saddle.

THE AMCHI'S VIEW OF MEDICINE

'Permit me to take this opportunity to tell you the history of our medicine,' he began in his quiet voice. 'It comes from a long, long time ago when the world was very different and men were purer in heart and nearer the gods than they are today. Before his fifth incarnation as the Prince Siddharta, the Buddha appeared on earth as the Buddha of Medicine. He taught the gods and the great sages and others ready for his wisdom. He brought his doctrine of healing from the realm of the immortals into the human world of India.

In time, many of the direct descendants of the Buddha's students arrived in Tibet. In the reign of our fifth King, Tron-sen-gampo, about 1300 years ago, two physicians came from India. They taught a woman to nurse her mother back to health, and when the king heard about it, he invited the strangers to his palace and placed them on thrones with nine jewelled cushions. One of these physicians married the king's daughter. Their son learnt how to read pulses, make medicines, bleed, order diet and heal by placing heat on the body's points of energy. It was the beginning of a long line of men who became the King's personal doctors.

The great Tron-sen-gampo also invited other men of medicine to a conference. One of his wives was a Buddhist princess from China. She also introduced medical treatises from her country and, because in those times, only men of noble birth could be physicians, she gave money to train twelve gifted students selected from all over Tibet.'

The tone of Nazir's voice and his manner of translating had changed: no longer the short, sharp phrases of an efficient guide, his sentences built a bridge from my world into the Amchi's near mythical realm.

'More information,' continued Sonam, 'came from Kashmir, Nepal, China and Persia.[1] Our nobles were sent off to the Chinese court for education, returning with a greater knowledge of astrology, pulse analysis and herbal remedies. Then, when the Mongols were converted to Buddhism seven hundred years ago, our medicine reached the farthest frontiers of our empire and our medical lamas were famous throughout Asia. Over the centuries we have had many scholar-saints. They left us their commentaries; some of them founded their own schools. We possess thousands of texts, but the all important ones belong to the ''Four Tantras'' I showed you in my room.'

Sonam gave us names of the wise men who chose and chose again to continue the work of past incarnations. Their genealogy provided an Ariadne's thread through the maze of colourful fables and magical transformations that he recounted with such pleasure. Historical exactitude was secondary. It was the spirit of the Buddha that had to be kept alive. Memory, in this instance, was more important than abstract reasoning, so from the mythical origins of Buddhist medicine, its history wove fact and fancy in a design threaded with the supernatural and natural which were distinguished only by the quality of experience.

Sonam was proud of the 'Four Tantras'. They hold information from Ayurvedic, Græco/Arab and Chinese sources adopted and developed by Tibetan sages. Nothing had been altered or added for near four hundred years.

Buddhism had made Tibet. Perched on top of the world, it was isolated in barbarism until the fourth century when Indian missionaries, tough and courageous, climbed through the Himalayas into a forbidding country roamed by untamed tribes with no written traditions or records of medicine. Sickness was fought with exorcism performed by Shamans whose hold over the people by magic and communication with the spirit world, was threatened by the new arrivals from a culture so far in advance of their own.

In tolerance, the Buddhists accepted many local customs and beliefs. From the seventh and eighth centuries, when the new doctrine, and thus its medicine, had taken root, Tibet was civilised and opened to an influx of new ideas from beyond its borders.

From India came the theory of the Elements and the Nopas. The Ayurvedic principles of diet, known to the Buddha, were modified from the torrid climes of the subcontinent, to suit local conditions. Persia contributed to remedies, and contact with China brought texts on astrology, a wider pharmacopeia and a more sophisticated method of pulse reading that, like the Nopas, was attuned to the turning planets and the seasons.

The Tibetans had rapidly knotted the strands of diverse medical knowledge into a synthesis still relevant to their social and religious needs today. In fact, this very advantage had petrified their medicine in the past, and Sonam was a living repository of a heritage that spanned thirteen centuries. And here was I, crouched on a mud floor in a timeless setting, a foreign representative of inevitable change.

In 1959, the Dalai Lama, followed by some 80 000 of his people, arrived in India, and Tibetan doctors had their first encounter with Western medicine. Their inductive, synthetic and intuitive art of healing came abruptly face to face with causal and analytical procedures. It was difficult to reconcile the two approaches. Sonam, in his journeys to the hospital in Leh, although impressed by surgery, had so far given no evidence of thinking his methods were outmoded. For how much longer would the likes of him continue practising their traditional medicine? Would Thelmy, grown to manhood, wear a robe, or might he take to jeans and shirt, use a thermometer and show a larger interest than his uncle in modern techniques? If so, he would most likely question many time-honoured beliefs and theories that, logical enough within their framework of Buddhist thought, contained elements of pure non-sense – such as letters placed on an infant's tongue to 'increase its intelligence'.

A THERAPEUTIC BATH

Seven children squatted in front of the Amchi. They had crept in to see foreigners and hear a good yarn. Their breath steamed out in the cold damp air, and Nazir reached over and drew the paraffin lamp closer. Positioning it, he manipulated his hands to cast shadows on the wall; birds, flowers, beasts, people, faces. The children clapped, and so did Sonam. Inevitably drawn into the fun, I invented dialogue and took part in the show, curling my fingers with the best of them.

Did I know a story? Could I sing Frère Jacques? What did it mean? I told Nazir who told Sonam who told the children. As for a story, I launched into Little Red Riding Hood. Instant success! Nazir, voice altered for each character, kept the children spellbound. The room became thick with smoke billowing in from the kitchen where a yak dung fire smouldered in the stove. Sonam got up, and we walked behind him. Thelmy, his second shadow, glided off to the soldier who sat next to a tin tub, chanting a mantra in preparation for his treatment. Sonam stood by, ready to scatter herbs into the water hauled over by three women. Steam married smoke in a veritable smog.

The Amchi in his stillness had a different kind of authority from the one we had encountered before. It came from professional poise coupled with long experience. His prayers were both committed and intense, and in the dirt and poverty of that farm kitchen, his presence radiated as if he were a messenger from the gods. The soldier stepped into the hip bath scented with herbs. The glow from the lamp threw huge shadows against the wall, the patient's face catching the light as it jutted turtle-like from his blanket. Whatever his motives, whether his faith sprang unchallenged from his youth, or came from mounting exasperation with western methods, his expression of a wounded animal eased into one of devout attention while Sonam invoked the Buddha's blessing.

As a stream of smoke stung my eyes. I no longer watched bemused by the quivering shadows and the movements that had captured me in a visual delight of mysteriously illuminated shapes. This unusual scene was ordinary in Ladakh, and the realisation jolted me out of my complacency. What on earth was I doing here, an untrained spectator on the fringe of an alien society. It was ridiculous to think I could achieve anything more than the superficial appreciation of the Amchi's work, easily understandable in its aims and self-evident gestures. I understood, but did I believe in the same power of prayer to the extent and even in the same way as the soldier? Obviously not. Moreover, I realised there was no way I could fool either myself or those around me that our differences would disappear.

Beneath the commonplace lay a sufficient doubt to make me feel an incompetent fraud. Somehow, I had to overcome my sense of estrangement by passing from my world into theirs or I would remain a pretentious voyeur. Even then, it was absurd to imagine I could become an instant Ladakhi. The only solution, was to try and link myself emotionally to the communal ritual, and in assuming a role of passive participation, initiate a non-verbal correspondence with the Amchi's teachings. With this in mind, I opened my heart, although I never spoke to him, then or afterwards, about my feelings of inadequacy.

Sonam prayed in a constant, steady monotone. Incantation is best learnt from a Lama since pitch and rhythm affect the vibrations surrounding the sick. The Tibetans illustrate chants by lines undulating across the parchment, the pattern unbroken by marks of timing. A priest gives life to the sacred text. But, if Sonam was not an ordained priest, his years in Karsha monastery had prepared him to chant a prayer. Besides, since any illness is the final expression of Ignorance, the mental and emotional links between doctor to patient are a vital aspect of a cure; a factor once so accepted that it is hardly mentioned by old-fashioned general practitioners, but now largely disregarded by contemporary medicine.

The soldier's eyes were glued to Sonam's face. The situation was a classic example of rational therapy tied to religion, and confirmed the Amchi's holistic approach to healing. At the end of the prayer, the family broke the circle around the soldier and Nazir and I went back to our room. Sonam soon joined us. 'The patient must sit in the water for twenty minutes,' he said, glancing at his watch, his only western possession other than his pen. 'Then, he will go to bed. We are just at the beginning of his treatment. His three Nopas, in particular the Phlegm, are upset from years of wrong food. I must change his diet, and have asked him to eat only well cooked food without any red peppers and spices, otherwise he will go on feeling listless and have a sweet/sour taste in his mouth. Poor man! In the army he took to Indian cooking like a leopard to a lamb. Do you have mineral waters in France?'

'Yes'

'So, French people lie in the water in those white baths I saw in Leh hospital?'

'Sometimes. It depends. In some places they have inside pools for everyone.'

'Our nomads in the high lands of Tibet would like that! Much easier than digging a hole in half frozen ground and lining it with a yak skin filled with hot stones and water. They always test the heat with their feet. After their bath, they wrap up in furs and drink hot yoghurt. Please tell me, do you bathe naked in France, or do you wear those short trousers I have seen on the trekkers?'

'People wear "bathing clothes", and the young women wear bikinis,' I answered, indicating the outline of the latter on my body.

'Oh yes! I have seen them on the girls when they go and lie in the sun by the river. They are very pretty.'

'The girls or the bikinis?'

'The girls,' said Sonam with a sweet smile, 'but do your doctors test the heart beat before putting patients into hot baths, and do they know the value of all the various kinds of mineral water as we do?'

'Yes. But not many of our doctors believe in their qualities. Hot springs in France are usually full of sulphur, but we also have mud baths and warm sea water cures.'

'Mud. Hm. Good. I have never seen the sea except in a photo an Indian friend showed me. I like to think about it.' Sonam sat down in the doorway, put his hands into his sleeves, and rocked forward onto his knees in a few moments of silence before continuing.

'We are careful with mineral waters because the body loses and absorbs properties through the skin and the flesh, right down to the bone. We call medicinal baths, "Lum"'[2]. He paused again. 'Ladakhis are not clean. It is sometimes the only way I can get old people to scrape off the dirt. You Europeans wash a lot, and I like the habit. Our "Lum" helps with paralysis, kidney and bile stones, old and aching wounds and water retention.'

'When are they dangerous?'

'If you have a fever, severe bruising or a loss of appetite. Our texts give details on the composition and the application of thermal waters. And we add ingredients to normal water when for instance, you suffer from nervous disorders and partial paralysis. We put in an infusion of musk or the dried dung of a musk animal, boiled for three days. Yeast is a substitute. Nazir, do you suffer from enlarged veins?'

'Not at present.'

'If you ever do, take a great heap of thyme, a small piece of fish and its bones and two big spoonfuls of strong beer and bicarbonate of soda. Boil the ingredients and add the distillation to your bath.'

'We started with our host's diet and have ended up in a fish bath,' I said to Nazir. 'Let's return to the Nopas. Please ask Sonam which of the Nopas are most troubled in this climate. Is it the Wind?'

'Not so,' replied Sonam. 'Our disorders are generally related to the Phlegm. I hear that Europeans have a predominance of Wind ailments. I know the Indians suffer Bile illnesses. It shows how our ways of thought and behaviour are different. But, it is quite natural for the Phlegm to govern the young, Bile the adult and Wind the aged.'

Each Nopa has its own symptoms which depend on the degree a Nopa's functions are augmented, diminished or completely overthrown.

'Are mental disorders also classified?'

'Indeed yes. They are grouped with illnesses caused by evil spirits. In all, we count 1616 illnesses. They arise from outer and inner causes such as seasonal change, poison, accidents, food, karma, way of life and evil spirits ... may your dreams be filled with good omens.' And with that he took up his saddle, smiled and left abruptly.

'They believe in that kind of thing here,' grunted Nazir opening his sleeping bag, 'the locals think they are forever being menaced, so don't go dreaming you're riding naked on a camel because that means death. Evil beings can inhabit a camel.'

Sleep, I replied, was also called the 'little death', and I was ready for it. 'I don't know what to think of Sonam,' I murmured, fighting fatigue. 'He is so disarming, so at ease with everyone. In the kitchen I couldn't take the bath therapy all that seriously, but there was such a strong rapport between the Amchi and the soldier. It was almost hypnotic. Do you think he is putting on an act for us?'

'I don't think so,' answered Nazir yawning loudly. I refrained from telling him that I had been relieved to leave the kitchen. It had needed no small effort on my part to break from personal interest into participation and actually project sympathetic feelings towards the Amchi and the soldier. I had had to forget I came from the West, and had become a human being with no past ... just someone present in a Ladakhi farmhouse at a time of healing. Although the concentration had drained me, it had been a marvellous release. The exercise of emotional identification had focussed not onto how but why Sonam, with his mystical orientation, accepted implicitly that invisible powers were essential in shaping the outcome of events.

My last thoughts before sleep were about my first trip East, to India and Nepal. I had been intrigued by the people's devotion to their god. Involving everyone from the ignorant to the learned, this capacity, as a blessing or a limitation, had vanished from the West. I was an intruder without the authority of either a doctor or an anthropologist. So much the better. I saw no point in categorising exotic cultures into a grid of reference drawn from our own society. A layman with no preconceived ideas, I embraced 'little death'.

NOTES

[1] Ladakh was most likely part of the Tibetan Empire by the eighth century AD. Its earliest monasteries were built in the first half of the eleventh century.

[2] Lum treatment is taken in spring and autumn, the times when the Phlegm (cool) and Wind (neutral) Nopas are at their crest and can be corrected through this therapy. Lum is not recommended for the Bile Nopa which carries the hot principle.

THREE

—————— • ——————

*Daily life with the Amchi—Local customs
and beliefs—The mixing of medicines—The
attributes needed for being a good doctor—The
theory and practice of pulse diagnosis*

A DAY WITH THE AMCHI

I awoke, and lying with my eyes closed, listened to the universal
sounds of a wailing child and a yapping dog. Chatter from the
kitchen, then the far away shout of a woman before she broke
into high throated song confirmed that I was in Ladakh. The smell
of damp, clay walls and rush matting made me sneeze.

Thick with sleep, Nazir and I stumbled into the kitchen. In the
corner behind the stove, we found the Amchi and Thelmy grinding
bark and roots on a stone slab. Sonam's bag, a fringed version
of the leather pouch carried by doctors, lay between them, brim
full of raw ingredients: mineral stones, twigs and pulverised plants
wrapped in pieces of white paper. A group of farmers came in
and sat next to him. In the conversation, their expressions passed
from concentration to pleasure. Eyes alight with love and respect
for their Amchi. His authority, after years in the monastery, was
absolute. He could read the sacred texts; his word was law. Born
in the district, Sonam shared the condition of his patients' lives.
Yet he was removed from them by his learning.

In that dark room furnished with a few rough wooden benches,
sacks of flour and sugar and a pile of rolled bedding, light from
a single window struck the copper of two, hand-held prayer wheels
lying on the wide sill. Their revolving drums were burnished from
generations of toil worn hands, for there was always time to turn
the wheel and propel a prayer to heaven. The great drums outside
Tibetan monasteries could hold almost a hundred million mantras,

and I never passed one without thinking of Isaac Newton. He too was convinced that prayers found their way to God by vibration; no passive request ever reached the Divine Ear.

The only other objects of beauty in the room were a battery of cooking pots, some appliqued with brass lotus design and all in good condition. In summer, visiting blacksmiths came round to make repairs and accept food eaten outside the house. A despised social class known as the Mons, they were probably the first inhabitants of the area to be converted to Buddhism between the third and fourth century.

Relaxed on the floor, we watched the grandmother prepare our tea. She knew we preferred it strong and plain unlike the Ladakhis who lace it with rancid butter or pink coloured bicarbonate of soda. After tea, the family, who had worked on the land since day break, moved out again without eating. Their meal would come later in the morning. The old woman completed her ritual sweeping of the floor, put her pots and pans on the stove, and sat back against the copper facing to feed a new born baby. I went over to cradle the child swaddled in a sheep skin, but she was reluctant to let her charge out of her arms. I asked why.

LOCAL CUSTOMS

'We must protect the new born from evil influence,' said the Amchi. 'When a baby comes into this world, it carries with it the merits and demerits of its past life. The vibrations around the infant are not stable. It must not be frightened and is kept in seclusion for the first month of its life. Festivals for well-wishing guests come later.' Sonam smiled. He bent down and passed his index finger lightly across the damp little forehead marked with a black vertical line that ran from the base of the nose to the baby's hairline. A sign of protection, it would be worn until the child was three or fives years of age. Amulets on its felt bonnet and silk neck cord shielded it from the evil eye and jealousy. Since Ladakhis believe that a boy is more precious than a girl, a male birth is kept secret, and for a while the baby is always referred to as a girl. Generally, all infants are called by names of a lower class, such as blacksmiths, to avoid arousing envy. This continues until after the harvest when the naming ceremony is conducted by a high ranking lama at a nearby monastery. With a simple benediction, the child is given a name carefully chosen for its meaning and the qualities it will bestow.

'Do you believe in demons?' I asked Sonam. He raised his eyes from the infant, and looking at me with a mischievous grin, replied, 'Everyone believes in things at the level of their understanding.' Popular religion in Ladakh comes from a sediment of ancient beliefs bound to Buddhism. Propitiation of the local nature deities and the devils who influence private lives and prosperity, join pre-Buddhist beliefs with priestly rites. During monastic ceremonies, votive offerings of millet flour and food used to lure and trap demons, are cast into fire. Goat and dog skulls hang on the walls of houses to deflect the potential anger of earth and sky spirits. Throughout the Himalayas, there are over 3000 different formulas for amulets.

Not wishing to embarrass the grandmother by staring too long at the baby, I moved over to the window. Nazir brought me a second mug of tea, this time lightened with the powdered milk used for the baby's bottle. Twentieth century food processing had found its place between pre-Buddhist superstitions and traditional medicine.

'Did you notice that small cylinder jar in the corner where the baby is sleeping?' asked Nazir. It was, he explained, used for another ancient rite of protection. At birth, the umbilical cord is cut with a knife. At the moment of separation from its mother, the infant's life force is guarded by an arrow, symbolic of the vital energy, that is placed head down in a jar filled with grain. This, say the Ladakhis, is the instant when the child receives the presence of its protective deity to keep its life force from being stolen away by evil spirits. I wanted to know more about the life force, so taking our tea, we moved over to where the Amchi sat with his patients, preparing remedies.

'We distinguish three aspects of the life force,' explained Sonam. 'First, there is the "rog", the core of vitality. The backbone of life or "rog" carries the "tsa". Like the prana of the Hindus and the chi of the Chinese, it is the energy that supports the third aspect known as the "lha" or the individual's consciousness. You can imagine the "lha" as a light radiating from the life force. These channels of life circulate through the body and the head and accompany the Wind Nopa. The "lha" moves to the gaps between the tendons of the hand from where it can extend outside the body and be captured by demons. That is why we press the thumb against the interior base of the third finger and block this passage from an invading demon, or against our own destructive emotions. The idea of the ''lha'' is older than Buddhism. It is the ''Wandering Soul'' known to the Shamans. The life force circulates through our bodies in a monthly cycle. If we decide to bleed a patient, we must take into account the position of the life force at the time of the operation. I wonder if your doctors know this? If not, even a simple operation can leave a patient in a sad condition if he is cut in an area where his vital energy has accumulated.'

Sonam went on to explain that the exchange of energy and information between our bodies and the exterior world is a continuous process for as long as we breathe. Nature's work goes on within and outside us. With all this cellular interaction one may wonder where our identity as individuals begins or ends. The skin covering our form is a semipermeable membrane capable of absorbing and expelling compounds and registering sensations. Perhaps we say an attitude is just skin deep in order to reassure ourselves that our real self has not been touched. Perhaps in the skin's reaction to a disquietening thought, we shiver, exclaiming, 'It gives me goose pimples.' Conversely, prolonged skin contact between loved ones is a physical act to attain emotional closeness. And, admitting that our inner being has been moved, we complain how he, she or it has got under our skin.

Sonam used the skin as a means of contacting the life force circulating in certain of the Wind Nopa's channels. He would seek to change a state of mind through massage with aromatics mixed with oil or butter to unblock these channels. Furthermore, through the skin, this interior Breath of Life was in direct communication with its exterior counterpart. For a moment, rather than having a profound sense of communion with Nature through my pores, I felt vulnerable. Ancient cultures saw Nature as 'a whistling wind tunnel of spirits'. In these terms, my skin was a sieve for prana that when diminished let infections penetrate my derma much as would a covey of lurking demons. My curiosity fired, I asked the Amchi how he decided if illness was caused by an evil spirit.

'One way is to test the urine,' he replied. 'The presence of an evil entity is seen by the urine's special discolouration and the patterns of its transformation during cooling. We call in a highly trained medical Lama for analysis. The process is repeated to avoid incorrect results.'

'Astrological influences, the person's profession or status in life, the Elements and the realms of gods and devils are all taken into account. Nothing happens by chance and every event is seen as a sign of something more significant that is happening around or within a human being. The urine is stirred, and four small sticks are placed in the form of a grid across the bowl. The cardinal points, with the South at the top, progress clockwise. The Elements follow the same pattern with Earth given the central position in the grid which has nine spaces indicating the patient's condition related to the surroundings. The position of the bubbles rising in the urine directs the Lama's opinion.

'Normal diagnosis is by smell, taste, colour, the quantity of steam and bubbles and the level at which albumen is formed, the amount of chyle and what the urine looks like when it is cooled. The results tell us which Nopas are out of balance and in consequence the type of sickness we have to deal with. For example, if chyle, an excretion of the blood, disintegrates without visible cause, it means there is an internal tumour.'

After pulse reading, urine analysis is the most important means of discovering and confirming the nature and location of disorders.[1] The procedure is uncomplicated, but it takes ten years to become an expert. When I asked about the symptoms provoked by evil entities, Sonam passed Thelmy a handful of roots[2] to grind, then gave his full attention to Nazir with his notebook.

'The third Tantra classifies the demonic powers that cause mental disturbances. In essence, they are the products of the three mental poisons. Each on the three realms, upper, middle and lower, has its own types of evil spirit. Those of the planetary spheres and those connected with the five Elements attack the nerves and the brain. We see their effects in epilepsy, convulsions and paralysis. Evil entities of the middle realm cause mental disturbance like depression and folly by entering the mystic channels that run from the ring finger to the heart chakra ... the seat of the life force. Demons from the lower realms are mostly ''Nagas'', half human, half water serpents. They can also inhabit toads, tortoises and yaks. Leprosy is one of their diseases, a karmic disease seeded from repetitive stupidity and harmful deeds.

'Please bear in mind that ours is a medicine of correspondence between the seen and unseen. Demons can dominate a weak mind, and we all have a part of our consciousness that corresponds to negative powers. They must be recognised and treated with medicines and prayer. The internal causes of all illness come from the mind and the results of karma. The external factors are seasonal change, food, poisons and evil spirits.

'In our texts, the word ''sin'' means a material organism. It can be a parasite or something so small that it is invisible. At this level, a sin is the material manifestation of a demonic power. Its presence can be recognised by the body's pulses . . . we will go into that another time.'

MIXING THE MEDICINE

Sonam grinned impishly and went back to mixing medicines with Thelmy. The boy, his bright squirrel eyes darting from face to face, had never stopped pulverising the ingredients between two grinding stones. Sonam took out a tattered notebook he kept for his observations on patients and the effects of the medicines he had mixed for different cases. 'Some herbs I can not get here. They are exchanged with other Amchis when we meet. I am now making up a compound for one of the men I saw this morning. Later, I will take you to visit my son in the monastery. Four times a year he comes with me into the mountains where we collect plants and minerals and he dries the leaves and roots in his cell.'

When the ingredients had been prepared, the Amchi added them to some melted butter and honey in a little water and stirred slowly. After the sticky liquid had cooled, he rolled the preparation into small balls. Tasting like toffee, they were easily preserved. One or two would be taken first thing in the morning on an empty stomach. The basis of this medicine, ideal for children, is known as the 'three horses'. For indigestion, Sonam used powdered pomegranate, black rock salt, ginger, piper nigrum and piper longum in a melted base.

We asked him how he measured the required amounts. He looked up and laughed. 'A good cook knows how to prepare a dish: a little bit of this, mixed with a little bit of that, but if he is a beginner, he measures all the time. I have been cooking for years!' But Sonam was only pulling our legs. Measurements start with a 'zho' equal to 10 grammes, then a 'shrang' (10 'zhos'). The largest is 10 'shrang'. The Amchi carried a long handled silver spoon that held an amount equivalent to a large pea. The Tibetan word for mix, he said, also means 'to produce remedies'.

The art of prescription lies in understanding the ingredients' correspondence to the five Elements. A medicine's taste indicates the quality of energy that will be released after digestion. Whether a formula should be 'hot' or 'cool' will depend upon the illness. In each case the Tantras lay down the exact procedure to be followed, even to the time at which the medicine should be administered. Much in these elegant theories goes way beyond the scope of everyday practice, yet the value of their prescriptions, gained over centuries of empirical observation, should not be underestimated.

Having completed their preparations, Thelmy replaced the grinding stones on the shelf above the stove, rolled up the bedding and trotted after Sonam. We were eager to follow him on his rounds, and our faces fell when he announced that the time had not yet come to leave the village. He still had to visit a family in the house next door; just a friendly call. Would we honour him with our presence?

A FRIENDLY CALL

'Just remember,' whispered Nazir, 'if we eat or drink, use the low, wooden tables and never place your bowl on the floor. It's bad manners. And, don't think you can stay with an empty bowl. The lady of the house will insist on filling it more than twice. Refrain politely after the third time. It's expected, but first swallow anything put in front of you.' He then wagged his finger furiously. 'Before you get smashed on chang, at least give the impression you know something about their ways, and sprinkle some upwards for the sky gods, horizontally for the earth gods and downwards for the nasties in the underworld.'

We followed Sonam to the house and climbed a flight of steps to the main door on the first floor. It was dimly lit by just one small window. An open fire smoked on a base of stones in the middle of the room, its light flickering across a worn rug on a low bed. Our host, a young farmer, had a wife many years his senior. A plain woman with buck teeth, she was ill at ease and hovered over the fire, hardly daring to look up. However, before serving tea and millet flour in metal bowls, she chanced a quick glance at us. We mixed the flour with liberal helpings of chang passed around by her husband and sat, backs against the bed, small tables at our sides, in the dense haze of smoke as we watched the Amchi talking with his friends.

The morning sun shone on his features, mobile in contrast to the blunt countenance of the farmer. Sonam listened, not once interrupting the man's solemn monologue. Then, with a slight, quick shift of his body, the Amchi changed the subject and drew us into the conversation. Two hours passed; our bowls were always replenished, and the woman, her manner less remote, offered a delicacy in our honour. She sliced off thin strips of blackened meat from a smoked leg of lamb. Fried with clarified butter in a pan that looked as if it had not been scraped since the Buddha was born, I trusted in the chang to roundly drown any 'sin', and accepted the first, sizzling morsel. At last she smiled, and raised her eyes to mine.

Floating on chang, we waited for the Amchi to make his move and leave. On request I took photographs of the couple. We were impressed by their dignity and stillness as they looked into the camera. Our farewells given, we departed behind Sonam. He was in high spirits. He had not treated any illness in that household, and I assumed our visit had been no more than a social call on

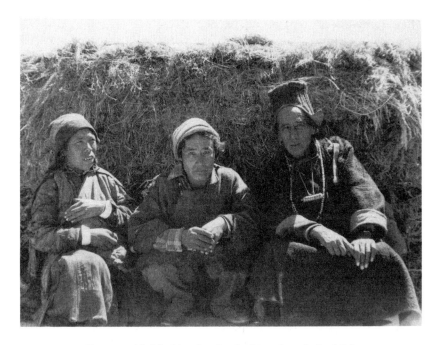

Sonam with his friends who had just lost their child

old friends. 'Our time there was very important,' said Sonam, halting in his stride. 'I did not want you to know the real reason or you would have entered with sad faces. Four days ago, they lost one of their two children through measles. I could have saved the boy had they called me earlier. The best remedy for such a loss is new company. Your presence has given them a subject of conversation that will last all winter. They will discuss what you were like, what you said, how you took photos, how you ate and how much you drank.'

THE ATTRIBUTES OF A GOOD AMCHI

As we walked along beside Sonam, I asked if psychology was part of an Amchi's training. Fingering the beads of his rosary, Sonam replied, 'You speak of human behaviour as if it belonged to a separate medicine. For us, its theme is always present. In the past few years I have had occasional contact with Europeans. I think it is difficult for you to tell the truth. You hide things from a doctor. But our folk talk openly. Remember the soldier so suspicious of you foreigners? If he had not felt he could confide his fears to me, my treatment could have been useless.

'In our training we are taught to contemplate the "Four Immeasurables", the four qualities essential to our practice. They are: immeasurable compassion, the wish for all beings to be separated from suffering and its causes; immeasurable joy, the wish for all beings to experience enlightenment and freedom from rebirth; finally, immeasurable impartiality, the wish for all beings to be regarded in the same light, not considering some as friends and others as enemies.

'My master, the Abbot, trained my intelligence and formed my attitudes,' said Sonam. 'A great Amchi absorbs more than information; his reason is acute and warmed by compassion when listening to his patients' dilemmas. He questions, reflects and often retires for meditation to clarify his intellect and senses before a diagnosis. Unless an Amchi acquires insight through meditation, the chain of events joining cause to effect, the seed into bloom, his outlook will not exceed the level of the sick whom he attends.'

Meditation nurtures intuition, and with intuition comes the merit of generosity. In the act of giving, no difference is seen between the giver and the receiver, and the Amchi gains wisdom. All acts are easily accomplished when motivated by generous compassion. An attitude rather than an emotion, compassion produces an assurance and a calmness recognised by the patient who, in this atmosphere of trust, finds no room left for an evasive or contrived response.

Nazir pulled me ahead before he spoke, more to himself than for my comments. 'It's that immeasurable impartiality that gets me. I find it very hard to take. Does it mean one mustn't even love or hate? My God! Imagine being impartial forever, sitting there beyond wants and needs and, in a way, beyond emotional commitment. The more I think of it, the more I feel this marvellous impartiality would leave me in a paralysis of perfection like a flame that no longer jumps as it burns.'

'Perhaps,' I replied, 'the Buddhists want impartiality, as Sonam has said, warmed by compassion. Still, their theory is very difficult to apply. We are all such egotists.' Although the Buddha taught that the mind rules the body, no lasting value is given to individuality in the Western sense. Buddhists are not concerned with the expression of individual capacity fulfilled by balancing the forces of Ego, Id and Super-ego. They believe man's progress depends on his efforts to detach himself from all desires. The Buddhists' truth is that suffering human beings are actually no-beings since they exist in a world of illusion.

> Where there is attachment, there is birth;
> where there is desire, there is attachment;
> where there is perception, there is desire;
> where there is contact, perception;
> where the organs of sense, contact;
> where the organisms, the organs of sense;
> where inclination derived from acts, incipient consciousness;
> where ignorance, inclinations.

Thus Ignorance is declared the root of suffering. Detachment leaves one without desire. Life is to be experienced with compassion for all sentient beings, here on earth and in other realms.

However, a great paradox remains. If life's conditions, including disease, are inexorably predetermined, from the earliest epoch of Ayurvedic medicine in India, doctors have chosen only to partially admit the validity of Karmic law. Otherwise they would lose the very meaning of their profession. Even if they accept sickness as Karmic retribution, it is their duty to re-establish physical and mental harmony. Even if the ultimate aim is spiritual development and the body impedes union with the divine . . . and moreover causes pain . . . a healthy mind in a sound physique can but speed man on his way aided by medicine, divine in origin.

The dry air filled my lungs and cleared the alcohol from my head. In this wide land, the sight of an unspoilt expanse was enough for me to relax and breathe deeply. Sonam's medicine, indeed a medicine of correspondence, had direct implications for my present mood. It was the space about me that I wished to draw within to afford a place for a change of outlook. Detachment seemed more attainable in this environment in comparison to the one I had left. Paris, with its garrulous shopkeepers, foul tempered taxi-drivers and indifferent, offhand professionals, frequently reduced me to a jelly of quivering fury, and incapable of rising above the situation, I fell into the trap of antipathy. I responded in kind to overt and covert aggression. Friends apart, most Parisians appeared to consider that generosity and kindness were best used as tools by people seeking favours from superiors. In short, the attitude espoused by most Parisians was: Be clever! Be wary! Eliminate your adversary with barbed wit and subtle innuendo! Above all, take no chances!

The Amchi had no idea of Western competitiveness yet in his meetings with Europeans he had noted a reluctance to speak openly. A Tibetan Lama at a Buddhist centre in France once mentioned his astonishment at the extent to which his students had a need of love. 'You are far more emotional than we are,' he had commented. He appreciated our social responsibility and respect for law and order, but laughed good naturedly at our tendency to intellectualise his teachings before summoning up the courage to experience and feel for ourselves the path of his instruction. At one seminar, he ruefully concluded by telling his flock to stop thinking. 'Anyway, you will soon forget everything I have said, so why don't you just go out and be kind to each other.' Upset by the demands of his lectures, put off by the discipline required in meditation and with ingrained habits of thought thoroughly dislodged, they spent the rest of the evening quarrelling and getting drunk. However, in the master's eyes, any short-term disruption to their psyches was of little importance. They had come into the Buddha's orbit in this life, and future incarnations would await their development. Detachment can be automatic, I thought, if we expand our sense of time.

PULSE DIAGNOSIS

But, time appeared to have stood still in the traditional scene about me. Farmers harvested the barley gathered into great bales transported on the womens' backs. They walked in single file alongside irrigation ditches that brought milky streams of water from the mountains shining in the sun. The road led us to a hamlet around a very small monastery. Sonam bade us to wait by the mani wall near a chorten and went off with his nephew to see if his patients were at home or still in the fields. Integrated into the landscape, mani walls are built from stones engraved with the prayer, 'Om mani padme hum'. This means 'Hail to the flower in the lotus'. 'Padme', the lotus, is a symbol for the chakras, subtle centres of mystic energy which can be coaxed into flower by breathing and meditation.

We settled down by the four foot wall and watched a woman approach. A child clutched her worn robe and dragged himself along with effort. She called out to Nazir in Urdu, asking when the Amchi would return, and throwing us a smile, cushioned herself on her sheepskin cloak against the stones on the opposite side of the dirt road. On Sonam's return from the village, he went straight to the woman. Without a word, he took the boy's wrists to feel his pulses. Sonam's hands became extentions of mind in direct communication with the child's disorder. He examined his tongue and eyes, and after a brief conversation, handed over a packet of medicine. The mother left without thanks or payment.

'What was the matter?' I asked Nazir who had gone over to watch the Amchi.

'Sonam said the body was dried out and that the regenerating Wind Nopa must be induced, anyway, the woman understood. She knows that the Nopas link the body to the universal powers.' Amazing, I thought, how the subtle powers of the cosmos flowed through that pathetic child afflicted with the miseries of some disorder detected primarily by holding his wrists for ten minutes[3].

'Please Sonam, tell us how you hear the pulses talk through your fingers,' I asked. He adjusted his hat, and pulling up his legs to cross them under his robe, began to explain.

'Once there was a very clever Amchi who attached a fine, silken thread to the wrist of a Chinese princess. Holding the thread, he accurately diagnosed her illness. I tell you this so that you can understand how extremely subtle the process is. Diet and behaviour react on the pulses, so neither the Amchi nor the patient should exercise themselves before a reading. No overeating, no mutton fat nor strong tea, chang, exposure to extreme temperatures, and no love making. Serious illness is best analysed at dawn on an empty stomach . . . a time when the Elements are at an equilibrium between night and day. The general Life Pulse is read on the cubital

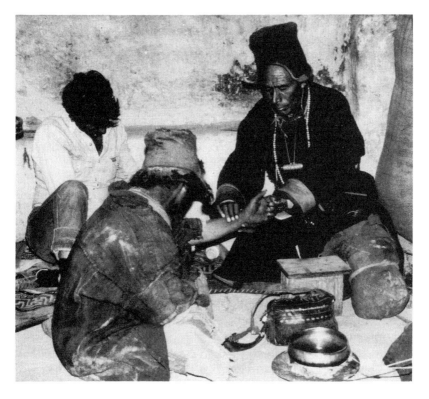

Sonam taking the Pulses

artery on the arch of the foot. It tells me a patient's life expectancy or the approach of imminent death.'

Sonam regarded me intently, the faintest of smiles hovering at the corners of his lips. 'I know nothing about your health, but perhaps you will permit me to read your pulses?' I offered him my right arm, he composed himself, and placed the first three fingers of his left hand on my wrist.

'Watch!' he commanded. 'I use my index, middle and ring finger of each hand, first with my left hand on your right wrist because you are a woman, then with my right hand on your left wrist. The procedure is the opposite for a man,[4] I read two pulses on the inner and outer side of each finger tip. The positions correspond to the twelve inner organs of the body. These we divide into five hollow organs and six full ones; twelve altogether, as we have two kidneys. On the right hand, starting with the index finger,

DIAGRAM OF THE PULSES

	Right Hand	Left Hand
Index Finger		
OUTER TIP	HEART	LUNGS
INNER TIP	COLON	SMALL INTESTINE
Middle Finger		
OUTER TIP	LIVER	GALL BLADDER
INNER TIP	GALL BLADDER	STOMACH
Ring Finger		
OUTER TIP	RIGHT KIDNEY	LEFT KIDNEY
INNER TIP	BLADDER	SEX ORGANS

I read the heart and the small intestines. On the middle finger, the spleen and the stomach. On the third finger, the left kidney and organs of sex.[5]

'With the left hand, in the same sequence, I read the lungs and large intestine, the liver and gall bladder, the kidneys and the bladder. Our classification of the organs into "Full" and "Hollow" ones comes from the Chinese concept of Yin and Yang, the double aspect of the cosmic life force known to them as "Chi".'

Tibetan medicine had taken much from the Chinese texts brought to the court in Lhasa during the seventh and eighth centuries. Spygmoly (pulse reading) is related to the seasons and a cyclic interpretation of the Five Elemets. Tibetans reverse some of the diagnostic positions used in China, The results, quite inexplicably, are just as satisfactory. Pulse reading depends on the skill of the physician in detecting impulses transmitted to the arteries and using them to diagnose factors causing disease. Impulses from the internal organs are carried in the flow of blood to the radial arteries which act as a go-between patient and doctor.[6] Each internal organ has its own system and is related to other parts of the body through the meridians of subtle energy.

Sonam, relaxed but concentrated, listened to the language of my Nopas bickering for the domination of my energy. He said I had a weak, cold stomach and was constipated most likely by the local diet. My general constitution was strong and had fine powers of recovery, but my heart had been damaged when young, and I had had difficult births. He was correct. Releasing my wrists, he continued. 'First, I find the patient's constitutional pulse. This gives me the temperament and thus the predominant Nopa. The pulse should beat five times during my respiratory cycle.

'There are three kinds of overall constitutional pulses: Male, Female and Neuter. These have nothing to do with the patient's sex. Each pulse, like those of the internal organs, varies in strength with the seasons, and we learn to decipher the thirteen basic pulses and their forty-seven qualities in diagnosis. The Male constitutional pulse is dominated by the Wind Nopa with its rough, thick beat, the Female pulse by the Bile Nopa and its rapid, thin beat, the Neuter pulse by the Phlegm Nopa's smooth, gentle and supple rhythm.'

Tibetans appreciate a poetic analogy to describe the pulse's qualities. The irregular death pulse is likened to a small bird caught by a vulture. The bird suddenly stops in mid flight, plunges, flutters and resumes its fall. For a mortal illness, the beat resembles a cow's wind-blown, drooling saliva. The beat of the heart taken on the wrist is as a voice shouting across open fields in the wind.

A DISCUSSION ABOUT HEALTH IN LADAKH

'Are you ever paid for your services?' I asked recalling Sonam's last consultation. He roared with laughter. 'Some thank me, sometimes. Others give me clothing or food, but few pay me.' There were doctors, he admitted, who demand fees before they touch a patient. He was not one of them, and the only money he counted on was a small monthly salary from the government.

'Are most of the doctors here like you?' enquired Nazir.

'I don't know if they are like me,' replied Sonam, 'but when the Dalai Lama visited Ladakh he called a census of Amchis. In all, at that time, there were forty, mostly here in the Zangskar; hardly enough for the country's 120 000 Buddhists.'

Health, he commented, was better now than it was ten years ago. The people had cut down on smoking intoxicating herbs, but government education had by no means eradicated the lack of hygiene. 'You have seen the conditions here. Poverty means filth. Education needs money and health needs food. It is a hard cycle to break in our surroundings.'

In the harsh Ladakh climate, overpopulation would be fatal and recently, infant mortality reached 50 per cent. At one time, polyandry controlled the number of births. The Amchi advised women to avoid pregnancy by keeping away from their men for two weeks from the first day of their menstruation. Babies were delivered by their grandmothers. In difficult cases Sonam showed them what to do, and had, on occasions used sheep intestines as gloves. He brewed herbs to relieve pain, and lately had been present at the birth of a 48 year-old woman's last child.

Sonam knew of plants to increase fertility.[7] Post childbirth pains were eased with poultices of mud from swallow or swift nests mixed with hot chang, or a dove's nest burnt on a fire composed of wood and sheep dung.

It was comfortable sitting against the mani wall in the sunlight freshened by a light, midday breeze. Sonam's patients were still out in the fields and he was in no hurry to move. Time to eat our chapattis, and, surely by no coincidence, a young monk ambled out of the monastery, his pleasant moon face beaming. He crouched down, offering us a handful of dried apricots taken from the pocket inside his robe. I noticed his hands. They were unexpectedly large with square tipped fingers smooth from lack of manual labour, and somehow out of place on his round, plump physique. The men chatted, and when the monk left, Nazir informed me that Sonam had a particular interest in the young man, the son of the rich farmer we were going to see. 'The Amchi tells me he has an awakened consciousness.'

'Then ask our Amchi how he judges the stage one has reached in inner growth,' I replied. Delighted by the question, Sonam settled down in front of us.

'We have four categories of consciousness,' he said with raised fingers. 'There are ordinary mortals born from the motivation of fear and desire. They have hardly any choice in the circumstances of their incarnation. Then, there is what we call ''The Universal Monach'', a person with a wider consciousness who can choose his birth but forgets what he had chosen for himself; the memory is lost. On the next level are those on their way to enlightenment; they have a degree of remembrance of past lives, whereas the enlightened ones are the ''Tulkus''. They can recall their previous existences and the entire process which brought them into this world.'

Our lecture was cut short as Thelmy bounded over the wall. The farmer, his family and others had finished work and expected the Amchi as soon as possible.

NOTES

[1] A disturbed Wind Nopa produces albumen that resembles goat hair. Albumen produced by the Bile Nopa tends to gather in the middle of the urine bowl. The Phlegm Nopa generates small, scattered particles of albumen. Mental disorders are indicated by an albumen sediment that resembles blue-white sand. Illness of a cool quality, resulting from imbalance in the Phlegm or Wind Nopa is indicated by transformation in the urine running from the side to the centre of the container. Illnesses of a hot nature that are caused by imbalance in the Bile Nopa are revealed by transformations occurring from the bottom to the top of the bowl. Urine from someone who is dying shows little variation, lacks colour, odour, bubbles, steam and taste.

[2] Four basic roots are mixed with other substances to purify the body's subtle channels. These are: *Angelica Sp, Asparagus racemosus, Polygonatum somnifera* and *Tribulus terrestis.*

[3] In 1976, Yeshi Donden, the personal doctor of the Dali Lama, visited an American hospital. He had prepared himself before arrival by bathing, fasting and prayer. After ritually taking the pulse of a patient, using his senses like a human electrocardiogram, he examined her urine in a wooden bowl. He spoke of winds flowing through her body, strange currents whose destructive energies ran in her blood. The cause, he claimed, came from the time before she was born when forces had opened doors that should have been kept closed. Now, her damaged heart could no longer cope with the stress that flooded her being. She suffered from congenital heart disease an interventricular septal defect which would end in heart failure.

Diagnosis rests on developing the senses to the highest pitch, especially the sense of touch by which the physician determines what imbalance has occurred in the body's energies.

[4] The organic representation of the female is the same as the male except that the position of the heart and lungs, read respectively on the right and left index fingers, are reversed for a woman. While the mystic entrance of the life force into her heart is oriented to the right, for men it is oriented to the left.

[5] Tibetan doctors, conforming to western physiology, speak of a pulse that is related to the genital organs. This pulse was originally considered to be the voice of the Samseu, a mythical organ of Sino–Tibetan origin situated in the lumbar region. The Samseu played an important role in forming menstrual blood, especially during the last 15 days of the month. It is a cosmic analogy to the waning moon, cool and white, which leaves the sun, hot, red and associated with blood, to predominate.

[6] Internal pulses are read from three segments of the radial artery on the left and right wrists. The median segment corresponds to the apophyse styloide. The distal segment lies between the median segment

and the thumb. The proximal segment extends from the median segment towards the elbow.

[7] *Plygonatum* leaves, Drynaria flowers and *Epyphyte Symplocos Ramosissima* fruit and bark were used respectively to increase or prolong fertility.

FOUR

⋅

*The Amchi treats patients in the house of a
rich farmer—The women of Ladakh—Sonam
discusses the Tibetan theory of conception,
reincarnation, diagnosis by proxy, the change
of sex in an embryo, and the constitution and
dissolution of the body*

A VISIT TO A RICH FARMER

Sonam led the way to a large, three-storied house. We walked
up high steps into the spacious salon. Judging from the modern
tanka on the wall, fine Chinese tables and rug, white cotton curtains
blowing in the open windows and brocade cushions, the residence
obviously belonged to a prosperous family. The top of the house
was partly covered by a flat roof, leaving the open area as a summer
kitchen. Half a dozen villagers and several children waited for the
Amchi in one corner. A particularly attractive young woman came
forward to greet us. On Sonam's introduction we shook hands,
sat down on reed mats and were handed bowls of tea with added
hot water poured from an embossed, long spouted kettle steaming
on the fire a few feet away.

Nazir followed the girl's every move. Aware of his attention,
she met his gaze openly, smiled and started a lively conversation.
Her behaviour confirmed the reputation that Ladakhi women have
an independence and a social and statutory equality with men
gained long before the days of the suffragettes. On the other hand,
equality involved work alongside their menfolk in the fields, and,
for the very poor, labour in road gangs.

'Don't you think Lobsang is beautiful?' asked Nazir in a low
voice. I agreed wholeheartedly. Her elegant black robe was belted
with a pink sash, and from her neck hung a thick, coral necklace

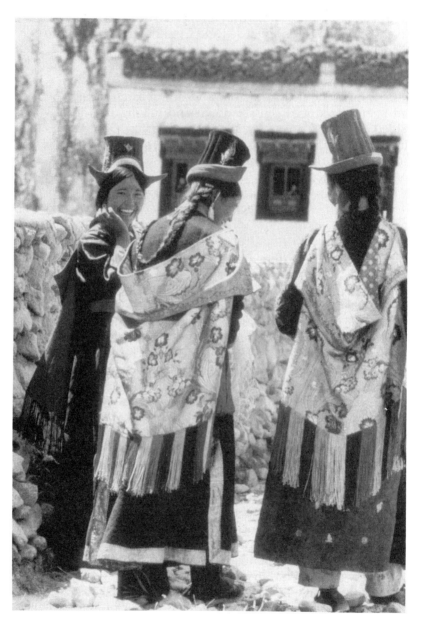

Dressed for the Harvest Festival, young beauties flash smiles attached to a delicately chaced silver and turquoise box containing some sacred relic or text. I was sure his intentions towards her were far from reserved. He grinned. 'Their ways are very strict, but in practice,' he said, 'they are pretty broad minded. They haven't any hang-ups about sex and I've known families who only let their daughter marry a man after they have had a child. That way they know that everything is in working order.'

The Amchi stood up to greet our host, a thin, small man whose white moustache dropped from a weatherbeaten face. When we had been introduced, he sat down and talking in a loud voice, gulped down six cups of tea in quick succession. Sonam then took him aside. Rather than take his pulses which would be far too active after work on the land and too much tea, he examined his fingers, severely knotted with arthritis.

'There are three different types of this affliction,' he said. 'One affects the bones, one attacks the nervous system and the last impedes the muscles. They all carry the same symptoms, but have a different pulse. I can cure each type with herbs provided they are not in active combination with each other. In another treatment, I place a small horn on the swelling and suck out the liquid without breaking the skin. I have been treating my friend here for two years now and, as you see, he is able to work again.'

For the next few minutes the Amchi questioned his patient and examined his tongue and eyes. The check-up completed, he left Thelmy to hand out packets of herbs and moved over to a pregnant woman.

Poised in concentration, Sonam felt the taut, or the slack, the high or the low, long empty, sliding, thin, rolling, dribbling or any other of the forty pulses possible that would indicate the condition of her internal organs. Each were entities in their own right. More than cogs in a biological machine, they were centres of activity governed by patterns of energy that yoked man to the universe. Sonam sat for ten minutes, head inclined, fingers recording and bearing witness to the mother's health and that of the developing child. Flesh on flesh, no cold metal was employed to test and measure life within the womb.

Tibetan anatomy embraces the physical and the metaphysical. The soul, synonymous with the life force, enters at the moment of conception to participate in the embryo's growth. Synchronised to the foetus' development, the mystic body invests the flesh with an anatomy of invisible channels and chakras that relay the energies of the three Nopas. The subtle channels often coincide with the network of blood vessels and nerve fibres to form a delicate ecosystem of the tangible and the intangible. Sonam made no distinction in the reality of the two anatomies. Their difference was one of function.

The Amchi seemed pleased with the woman's condition. Thelmy, as usual, sat cross-legged next to him, devoted and attentive. The texts warn against secrets divulged to an unsuitable student whose mind, like an inverted pot, refused to hear or understand. Nor should he be a leaky pot that forgets everything; let alone a defiled pot with a mind impure from wrong motives and filled with preconceived ideas. Sonam's nephew was a sound, pure receptacle.

The next patient, an old woman, had swollen eyes and gums almost bloodless with the 'Pale Malady', anaemia. Sonam took her pulses. Her diet, he said, was to include mutton, fresh butter and yoghurt, no fish, no pork and nothing with a bitter taste. The Amchi gave her a mixture of herbs based on Swertia Chirata to be taken with butter. This evening he would prepare medicines and an emetic. 'I may have to give her a purgative next time. It depends if her condition is at its peak or not. Too strong a medicine or therapy too soon is as powerless as too little, too late. The illness comes from a bad diet. Wrong food makes bad blood. But a correct diet,' he continued, 'is in harmony with the seasons and the condition of the Nopas. When food is correctly digested by the Nopas' action in the stomach, it is transformed into the "Seven Bodily Constituents": blood, muscle, fat, bone marrow, seminal fluids and menstrual blood. With a change of diet, it takes a week for a man's semen to alter in consistency and smell. These seven constituents sustain the body's development but are weakened if the Nopas' digestive actions are out of balance. Ideally, after a meal, the stomach should hold one third solids, one third liquid with one third remaining empty.

I reflected on the obesity I had come across in America. Paunches jiggled over young men's trousers; fat women waddled around supermarkets; over-coloured, processed food irritated the eye in banal commercials; sugar seeped into everything edible. Two hundred years ago the annual consumption of sugar was seven and a half pounds per person per year. Average consumption in the USA is now more than a hundred pounds a year.

Our bodies reflect the food we eat. Although we have little choice in our constitution, we certainly can have a say in the quality and the quantity of the stuff that we feed to our flesh and our blood, to our bones and our skin. I once came across a pop-psychology quiz in a women's magazine. It offered a choice of menu by which the reader revealed her character. Compatible lovers were suggested by further tests. Definitely not to be recommended was the type who fancied pigs trotters and intestines, whereas gentlemen salivating for sweet desserts and pretty ice creams won the day. They are the suitably soft hearted good guys. The choice is ours. We can buy food for health or adhere to the promptings of the junk food and fizzy drink industry and become overfed, undernourished slobs.

'UKPA' TREATMENT

A nervous teenager knelt in front of the Amchi. The boy had been treated for convulsions since childhood. After examining his eyes, tongue and pulses, Sonam took a spiral-topped gold needle and wound dried Gebera leaves round its head. Lighting it, he placed the needle half a thumb's length from the Brahma point at the very centre of the crown of the boy's head.

'This is "Ukpa" treatment,' he announced. 'It is a light heat therapy to reorganise the disturbed Wind Nopa whose channels activate the senses and protect the brain.[1] In this case, a demon has upset the life force in his Wind Nopa. Prayers and rituals directed by the Lamas work with my treatment in healing him. He has fewer attacks. As you may have noticed, I placed the needle slightly away from the crown point because the boy is still young and the direct heat could be harmful. Alternative positions are seventh neck and the fourth dorsal vertebrae.'

Ukpa is not to be confused with acupuncture. Although many of the meridians are similar, it is given with rigid needles applied to seventy-one points on the body, limbs and head. Different needles are used to achieve different effects. Silver dispels mucus, copper dries out what Sonam termed 'mucus-blood' and gold is used for the nervous system.

In heat therapy, metal, wood, stones and compresses made from herbs or bird droppings are laid on the surface areas connected with the neutral Wind and cool Phlegm channels. The areas connected with the Bile channel are never used because of its hot nature which would only be increased and disturbed by any form of heat. The principle that opposites pacify and restore equilibrium is used in diet as well as in medicines and behaviour.

In a charming counsel, Tantra texts announce that 'People who suffer from an imbalanced Wind Nopa, whose food has been heavy, who live in a cold climate and have been upset by rude, noisy companions, should recuperate in a warm valley protected from winds, eat lightly and converse with gentle friends.' Substitute 'urban stress' for 'companions' and I, by serendipity, was following precisely that advice.

The Amchi welcomed each patient and encouraged them to answer his questions at length, or in an easy silence attended to diagnosis. No one hurried. Sickness had its place in life and was a condition natural to this world.

'Your apprentice clearly knows his job!' I said, as Thelmy handed out a packet to an old man.

'Oh that! Yes, the boy is quite reliable. That powder is a well known home cure. It's made from nutmeg and coriander seeds. The old folk use it in hot oil compresses to ease aches and pains brought on by the Wind Nopa.'

SONAM THE SURGEON

A peasant, well past his prime, walked over to the Amchi. With furrowed face, curved back and hang-dog expression, he seemed to carry the world's miseries on his narrow shoulders. He sat down and bared his torso, complaining of a pain behind his left shoulder blade. Sonam fingered the slight swelling saying, 'It is not so sore, is it? You made no movement when I touched you, so why the sad face? Come on, Jigmy, what is the real problem?'

Jigmy's expression turned to a grimace. In fits and starts he wailed his tale of woe. Nazir, head bowed and hand across his mouth, did his best to keep a straight face. 'He's asking the Amchi for an aphrodisiac, a very strong one, and this time he's prepared to pay in cash.'

Sonam asked the old man if he had just taken on a nubile young wife. Poor Jigmy could barely get his words out. 'My wife,' he wheezed, 'as you well know, is no spring chicken, but I want to keep her for myself. Now she's gone barmy over her young cousin just back from Leh. He's bone idle, just flops about the house and does no work. All he wants to do is jump my woman in the morning and count the goats with her at night. She must have bewitched him with a love philtre from the Shaman.'

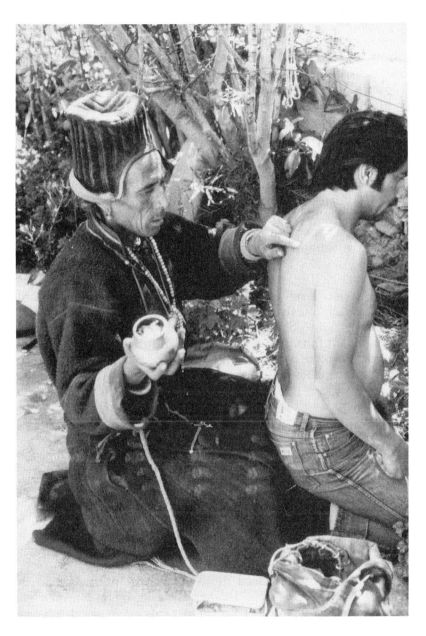

Sonam demonstrates on Nazir the cupping he performed on Jigmy, who refused to be photographed!

Despite the Amchi telling him that an aphrodisiac wouldn't get his wife back and that the lover wouldn't stay forever, Jigmy asked for a magic love potion. Sonam refused. Those things, he insisted, were the Shaman's business, not his. While the dejected fellow rattled on in evident distress, Sonam took a dried fruit from a Terminala Cherula bush and set light to it in a small, copper bowl. He placed the heated bowl four fingers width to the right of the swelling and left it there for the next 45 minutes to withdraw the congestion.

Some swellings are formed by undigested food that produces unhealthy blood. Others come from old wounds, worms in the flesh or too much humidity. Internally, they can be detected by pulse, a particular thin, weak beat, or from urine samples that contain bubbles resembling fish eyes. Back hunched, the bowl sucked tight to his skin, old Jigmy looked the total victim.

Sonam beckoned us close and showed us two more instruments for heat treatment. One was a metal rod bent at one end with a wooden handle. The other was a metal plate pierced with well-crafted holes. 'If massage, hot baths and compresses don't work, I have to use stronger methods.' he said. 'I heat this rod until it is white-hot; like that, it causes less pain. Then I guide it through these holes to the points on the spine that correspond to the internal organs I want to treat. I also use the iron rod to cauterise infected wounds. Another strong therapy is blood letting. We prescribe it for fevers and blood disorders.'

BLOOD LETTING

In Oman I had once watched an Indian doctor in a desert clinic giving a deep injection to an unflinching Bedu woman. Her fortitude, and even desire for injections, in his opinion, came from the association of pain with healing; a cultural imprint common to traditional medicines.

'I gather you are experts in bleeding. Will you be doing any today?' asked Nazir, feigning detachment, for I knew he hated the sight of blood.

'Blood letting is practised more among the nomads than the farmers,' Sonam replied. 'Nomads eat a lot of mutton and yak meat with great helpings of butter. This causes high blood pressure. If you wish, I can bleed you straight away. It will relieve the congestion I have noted under your eyes.'

Nazir winched in alarm. But, surrounded by curious farmers, he obeyed Sonam's gesture, and went over to the doctor's mat. The Amchi pressed the pouches under Nazir's eyes, and taking a small scalpel of polished bone, he washed it under boiling water from the kettle. Pinching the bridge of Nazir's nose, he pricked the cartilage between the nostrils. One large drop of blood oozed out and down onto Nazir's moustache. 'There!' You will note the difference tomorrow. Now, how about some tea?' Sonam handed him a cup delivered by Thelmy, always half a jump ahead. 'We have the maxim: after fire treatment, dance. After bleeding, stay as immobile as yoghurt. Be thankful you are just having tea instead of boiled sheep's blood with barley and salt. That is what we give to patients after severe blood letting or haemorrhage.'

'Honoured Amchi,' pleaded Nazir, 'in the name of compassion, please stop talking about blood or I will faint.'

'If you do,' Sonam replied in a deliberate provocation that made our audience bray with laughter, 'I will have to bleed you again, this time from the bridge of the nose.'

Sonam rarely resorted to such therapy. He thought it dangerous despite his knowledge of the seventy-one points he had studied on his master's diagrams. His medical Lama, trained in Lhasa, had had considerable experience with the 'dob-dob', monks who were keener on sport than study. They would leap from the second storey of their monastery onto piles of sand in a pastime they found much more fun than raising their consciousness. The game increased their blood pressure already high from a diet of salted tea, yak butter and barley porridge. At that altitude, shock and pressure from accidents soon left these athletes in need of bleeding.

Two or three days before treatment, said the Amchi, the patient takes a preparation which separates healthy from unhealthy blood and prevents the loss of essential elements. Diseased blood shows little balls which, in the light, reflect rainbows or the shape of a feather. Another variety appears with lines in it. 'We have to be careful. There are so many things to take into account; the state of the patient, the type of illness. We must be exact in the choice of point and time for letting blood. I am not expert enough,' concluded Sonam.

He recalled an Amchi he had known as a child. A wild character and ugly as a toad, this man practised in the mountains near a thermal spring. He bled people in spring and autumn when they came for medicinal baths. Shouting and singing, he would hustle up to thirty patients into a line, take their pulses in a cursory fashion, and tie tourniquets on their arms before making incisions with a fist full of instruments. He always demanded payment in chang. 'I was amazed,' said Sonam, chuckling, 'because none of his patients were ever the worse for wear, but he, hooting drunk and covered in cuts and bruises, would gallop off across the stones. He went on letting blood, drinking and falling off his horse until too old to move.'

As Lobsang left the roof, Nazir excused himself and followed. A little later, I too went downstairs to the ground floor. After the bright light outside, I failed to notice the lady of the house in the semi-darkness. A good looking woman, she called out, came over to take my arm, and talking in a confidential tone that implied we had no language barrier, ushered me to an alcove prepared with bedding on the floor. The arrangement was far more luxurious than my previous night's accommodation. I thanked her and then went out for a stroll.

As I walked along I mulled over Sonam's techniques, I recalled a discussion I had had at Leh hospital with a Ladakhi doctor trained in Srinagar.

'I am all for our traditional Amchis,' he had said, 'they fulfil a basic need in a simple and inexpensive way. We have not enough doctors or clinics here. When they are good, their diagnosis is good. They can arrest certain cancers in their early stages, but then we don't have much cancer in Ladakh.' Our walk along the corridor took us to the operating theatre.

'It may not look all that well sterilised to you, but post-operative infections are rare in this hospital. Wounds heal fast in the dry climate and the altitude helps with increased ultra-violet radiation. All the same, don't let an Amchi operate on you. Surgery, Tibetan style, is not advised.'

A call had brought our tour to an end, and I left not knowing whether he was Buddhist, Moslem or a Christian from the Moravian mission in Leh.

DIAGNOSIS BY PROXY

I came across a track which led me past barley fields rippled by the afternoon wind. On coming to the river, I heard high-pitched screams and saw Lobsang running off with her head and shoulders covered in white foam. Nazir, in hot pursuit, towel in hand, attempted to wipe away the overdose of shampoo given in his efforts at courtship. I turned back to the village.

It was restful to be alone. In my shifting thoughts, I found comfort in the rocky permanence of the landscape and the indifference of geological time to the desires of man. I, for one, was not ready to eliminate them from my mind. In this incarnation I coveted love for life and all that it implies: laughter and the give and take that guarantees rich relationships; the excitement of great music, works of art that draw dreams from my heart; the satisfaction of work well done and the host of other first degree wants undistinguished from needs. Sonam's devotion to his profession and his faith carried him forever onward to the goal of ultimate perfection, but I had no unlimited horizons. We were, in my view, all imperfect creatures of an imperfect creation, and our pretence of understanding absolutes was no more than the conceit of a limited intelligence.

Just short of the house, a dust-covered woman trotted briskly by on a pony lathered in sweat. It was unusual for anyone to be in such a hurry, and my curiosity increased as she rode into the courtyard. Ever-ready Thelmy clattered down the exterior stairs to help her dismount. I followed them into the kitchen at a polite distance. The traveller headed straight for our hostess. They embraced warmly before the woman knelt in front of the Amchi and exchanged a few words. Sonam smiled and nodded his head reassuringly. She stood up, took off her fine Parak, a head-dress of turquoises, pearls, and coral beads, and washed her hands and face. She then settled down to eat curds from a silver bowl and drink tea from a tin mug.

I rested in my corner until our hostess called me for tea and an introduction that left the visitor informed but myself still ignorant. Both women had glorious smiles. I could hardly contain my impatience for Nazir's return. Finally, he came in with Lobsang; they were on cloud nine. I wanted to catch his eye, but the rascal, mug in hand, chatted with the women for what seemed like a month of wet Sundays. I was left to dampen my curiosity with the contents of my notes. At last he ambled towards me.

'So!. What do you think has been going on?' he began.

'Lobsang got soap in her eyes,' I replied curtly. He snorted and lit a cigarette.

'As for what's going on here,' I continued, 'I'll give you an uneducated guess. The guest is a relative, perhaps a sister of our hostess. She galloped here to bring some news which can't be too serious since no one is crying. Now tell me, what really happened?'

'Well,' answered Nazir exhaling a perfect spiral of smoke, 'your

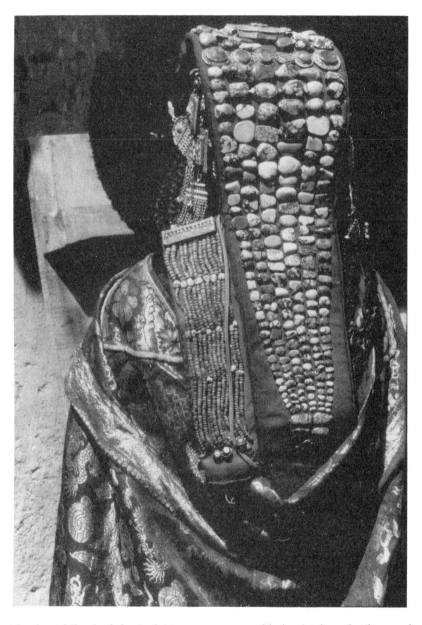

The famed *Parak* of the Ladaki women, a portable bank of coral, silver and turquoise

miss is as good as a mile. The woman is, in fact, a cousin.'
'Why does she want to see the Amchi, she looks quite fit?'
'Hold on! I'm coming to that. Now listen to this. She wants
Sonam to take her pulses tomorrow morning, after a good night's
sleep, so that he can find out what's the matter with her daughter.
The child is very sick and can't travel.'

'So Sonam takes the mother's pulses to diagnose the daughter's
illness,' I said.

'That's right. Diagnosis by proxy. It all sounds a bit like fortune
telling doesn't it?' Nazir's grin faded as he pulled on his cigarette.
'There's good reason why the Amchis do this. Diagnosis by proxy
is an old Chinese practice. Doctors in China used to be paid to
keep their patients well. Bad health meant a bad doctor, so any
way of knowing if an illness could be fatal or incurable gave the
doctor a degree of self-protection. To be forewarned is to be
forearmed and he could then decide what action to take.'

Diagnosis by proxy was just as logical to the Tibetans. All beings
have their own portion of the life force, a factor that can be touched
and detected by the same principle in others, either through har-
monic resonance or by shared influence.

Later, after the visitor had retired and the family, busy in their
talk, gathered around the stove, Sonam, laden with three bowls
of chang, made himself comfortable between us.

'Saloo!' he said unexpectedly as he raised his drink, adding in
English, 'French trekkers' to explain the toast. Sonam looked at
us expectantly, one hand fingering his beads. He waited for Nazir
to ask the first question. It was about pulse divination, which did
not surprise him.

PULSE DIVINATION

The Elements, said the Amchi, support life and thread us together,
but we and they are subject to time and to change. In a seasonal
procession, each Element gives a predominant pulse to five of the
internal organs. This association of Element and organ is read in
a pattern of relationships from which the future is predicted.

The Elements used for pulse divination are those of traditional
Chinese medicine: Fire, Earth, Metal, Water and Wood. Fire gives
birth to ash or Earth. Earth contains minerals or metal that provokes
the condensation seen on the outside of a metal cup filled with
water. Water gives rise to vegetation or Wood and Wood feeds

Fire. Such is the generative or friendly-parent cycle, leaving Fire to be the enemy of Metal (it bends it), Wood, the foe of Earth (it saps it), Earth, of Water (it obstructs it), Water of Fire (it kills it). Each season has its predominant pulse: Spring for the liver (Wood), Summer for the heart (Fire), Autumn for the lungs (Metal), and Winter for the kidneys (Water). The spleen (Earth) pulse is given the last 18 days of each season. The pulses are either friendly or antagonistic in their relationships.

'To give you an idea,' continued Sonam,' a healthy person in spring should have a predominant liver/Wood pulse. If we find the kidney/Water pulse is abnormally strong, the symptoms will effect the mother or father of the patient because Water is the parent of Wood. If the lung/Metal pulse is abnormal, its symptoms will apply to an enemy of the patient since metal is the enemy of Wood.

In a healthy person, the predominance of an unseasonable pulse and its favourable or unfavourable alliance with the other organs, an Amchi can predict future events. Information comes from what they call the 'Seven Astonishing Pulses'. These indicate household conditions, movements of relatives, the strength or weakness of an enemy, financial matters, directions from where harmful influences might come, the outcome of an illness diagnosed by proxy, and whether the child of a pregnant woman will bring honour to its family.

Omens too can play a part in prognosis since invisible powers lie behind everything that happens. Events, in partnership with the supernatural, reveal the quality of the unseen world. According to the texts: if the messenger sent to an Amchi is a monk, the case is favourable, but should the messenger arrive on a donkey, camel or buffalo and wear a red flower, carry a stick or a weapon, it indicates that the patient will die. If an Amchi on his journey to a sick person comes across a heap of grain, a pretty woman carrying a child, a bucket filled with curd, or hears the sound of bells, all will be well.

Traditional Eastern medicine relies on a multitude of observations taken from natural events and their possible relevance to illness. Today's epidemiologists seek reasons for cot deaths by methods that are not far removed from those of ancient China. In determining causes for sudden infant deaths, relevant data ranges from the time of day or night that babies die, the seasonal temperature, the day of the week and where they were born, to whether their parents were married or not, race, sex and age of mothers etc.

Statistics give results. So why not ask if a pregnant woman had encountered a fire engine when crossing the road or had been frightened by a jet flying low overhead? Modern substitutes for the proverbial buffalo menacing her path, or an inopportune crow croaking its message of doom.

'If you remember,' continued the Amchi, 'I spoke of the three types of pulse: Male, Female and Neuter. We can also use them to interpret omens. If a man has a Female pulse, we say he will live long. If a woman has a Male pulse, we say she will have many sons. If she has a Neuter pulse she may well have no children. Often people with a Neuter pulse have enemies in their family but good friends in high positions help them in difficult times.' He paused and raised his hand. 'The Neuter pulse can also belong to an evolved one: a teacher or holy man destined to help others.'

I asked if the monk who had eaten with us by the mani wall had a Neuter pulse. 'Yes,' he replied with no further comment. With that, Sonam rose and retired with Thelmy to the other side of the room. Our host stomped in from the fields, Lobsang and the visitor came down from upstairs and together we warmed ourselves near the stove where our hostess was boiling noodles. Night came. As I watched Thelmy bring a lamp to his uncle, I realised that I had forgotten an important question. Did a blood relative give a better proxy reading than a wife or a devoted friend?

The truest link of all, said Sonam, is love.

We left uncle and nephew to discuss the day's work. In the simplicity and hardship of their lives, the Amchi was instilling in Thelmy a healthy respect for the web of existence. Every day, he absorbed advice given to patients on the interaction between behaviour, a state of mind and health, between food and medicines and the chain of reactions that passed between the physical and subtle anatomy channelling us to the universal Elements, the precursors of our environment.

BIOLOGICAL CONSCIOUSNESS

Jung would have understood, for he thought that coincidence is often too remarkable to be explained away by chance. He accepted the existence of a cosmic force that worked within its own laws. He called this phenomena of chance synchronicity.

Later, the English physicist professor David Bohm proved that some coincidences are not entirely random. Using bursts of protons and other sub-atomic particles, the path of one was found to directly influence the path of another, thus demonstrating 'action at a distance' – a controversy that had long occupied the minds of physicists.

On the level of cellular communication, one theory proposes that a single cell, from which our bodies evolved, was fertilised when lightning – the divine thunderbolt of the Buddhists – struck through the methane mists of a cooling earth and life began. Under a cloak of diversity lies the uniformity of plant and animal enzymes. The interrelated facets of evolution are even apparent in our own cells. In our bodies we harbour the heritage of a biological past we share with every animate form. Nature's biochemical interactions regulate all movement from microscopic organisms to man.

Alas, we are not in direct communication with our cells which already possess their own consciousness. While we rely on machines, they, more likely, share a direct biochemical language of their own that might well underlie the recorded instances when girls, living together in dormitories, are prone to spontaneously synchonise their menstrual cycles.

Another form of biological consciousness was demonstrated in the early seventies when L. G. Lawrence, an electrical engineer in California, made experiments with plants aligned to the constellation of Ursa Major. He discovered they received 'deep harmonious oscillations' from outer space through their biological sensors. As Lawrence had no such sensors in his equipment, he could not decode the signs. 'I don't believe,' he wrote, 'they are directed at earthlings. I think we are dealing with transmissions between peer groups, and because we don't know anything about biological communication, we are simply excluded from these communications.' The signals were, apparently, beyond the known electromagnetic spectrum.

In his particular way, Sonam was teaching Thelmy to interpret the voices of the universe singing through the body's biology. It brought to mind a clear winter's night when a small boy, all of four years old, had negotiated the stairs to grab his grandfather's hand. 'Come call the stars to sing to me!' he had cried, eager to have their night-long chorus fill his ears. For him, those high, glinting orbs were no silent objects. They were living beings waiting to be contacted for his pleasure.

Poets, mystics and children retain the ancient ability to identity with an object or person through intuitive perception that eliminates any difference between subject and object. In pulse prognosis, Sonam incorporated this intuitive identification with a strict discipline of interpretation. Used as divination or in diagnosis, it came from centuries of observation organised into a medical philosophy that absorbed both rational and irrational factors.

In the shadow of my alcove, I reflected on identification. I pictured my body encompassing the heavens, yet I could not imagine what it might be like if I were touched by the forces of the primeval Elements. Their raw power, I thought, would surely disintegrate me. Little wonder that the ancients recognised great hierarchies of gods and devils acting as intermediaries, their names changing with their function in the constant process of growth, decay and eternal renewal.

'You look pensive.' came Nazir's voice. 'It's time to eat, so come and join us.'

A meal of tsampa and noodles with chicken and chang, left me licking my fingers. I sat with the family in the womb-warmth of the room, relaxed and happy to hear them talk in the dim light. The meal concluded, I withdrew to my alcove. Out of the murmuring, Nazir's voice soared in an Urdu ballad, and lulled to the edge of sleep by the haunting song, I curled up under quilts smelling of dust.

EMBRYONIC SEX CHANGES

Thelmy woke me at dawn. Abominably bright for such an hour, he babbled away in his cracked voice with his face close to mine in utter disregard for my lack of comprehension. He was such a delightful little squirrel that I hugged him. Taking my hand, he pulled me from the covers and stiff from sleep, I joined Nazir for tea.

'Morning!' he greeted. 'Thought you'd better wake up and be ready for Sonam. He's upstairs prognosing. Here, take some of these corn cakes; they're delicious, and we have condensed milk as well.' Lobsang sang as she placed handfuls of dried apricots in a cloth ready for the departure of her mother's cousin.

Once we had waved the cousin on her way, the lady of the house told Sonam to sit down and have a bowl of fresh yoghurt. She was a woman used to being obeyed, and he, with the air of a schoolboy caught in the act of truancy, squatted down meekly.

He was an excellent actor when the occasion warranted him playing a certain role.

When we questioned the Amchi about the visitor's child, he was not at all happy. The girl had pneumonia and a high fever. Although he foresaw her recovery and had given medicines and instructions for her care, he expected complications would come later and intended to make the three day journey to her village in a week's time. 'There are bad influences nearby,' he mumbled to himself, spooning down the yoghurt. 'The Shaman there meddles with evil forces.' He quickly changed the subject, and with a happier expression said, 'But, I am pleased to tell you that the lady is two months pregnant and her child will bring honour to the family.'

We asked him if he could predict the baby's sex. 'Yes I can. First, by the pulse. A mother's right kidney pulse, when strong, means a boy; the left kidney, a girl. A boy usually lies to the right side of the belly, a girl to the left. Also, we can change the child's sex with medicines, but it only works with a female embryo, and must be done within two and a half months from conception. Other ways are mentioned in our texts. We employ effigies made of a special metal, and perform Tantric rites under specific astronomical conditions.' He fell silent again, reluctant to speak of details that we might scorn as nonsense. From the supernatural, he turned to medical information.

'If conception takes place on the 4th, 6th, 8th, 10th and 12th day after the menstrual cycle, the baby is a boy. Odd dates mean a girl,' he continued. 'A being is drawn into incarnation by desire; the strongest attraction back into this world. If the consciousness of the child-to-be identifies with the mother at the time its parents are making love, the incarnation will be in a male body, when the attraction is for the father, a female.'

'It all sounds very Oedipal to me,' I remarked to Nazir. Sonam wanted to know what I had said and was intrigued by our explanation. The Greek tale was enough. Freud was ignored. 'Yes, we too could say that when a "wandering soul" is drawn towards, and desires the mother, it wants to be in the father's place and know her love, and so it incarnates as a boy.'

So we choose our parents!

Applied to myself the reason was far from clear. I was indifferent to both my mother and father. Why had I been attracted to them in the first place? My mother, a spoilt, self-centred but charismatic woman, had never been interested in children. In her second pregnancy, she rashly promised her apparently barren and unhappily married elder sister a baby if she produced twins. Even during labour, the doctor had not detected my presence, and my birth was a second shock after I had pushed out my twin sister, born deep blue and near strangled with the cord around her neck. The sight of this dark child sent our maternal grandmother reeling to the floor, horrified by the prospect that her son-in-law possessed recessive negro genes, or, just as unsavoury to this South African 'grande dame', that her own ancestry might be polluted by black blood. In the tumult, my arrival was hardly welcome.

My Aunt took me home with her. She remarried, and when I was six, she and my stepfather told me of my biological parents. Since I had always known my aunt as mother, and my true mother, father and sisters as aunt, uncle and cousins, their new status made no emotional sense. Alienation from my adopted parents came only at the age of ten after my mother/aunt conceived her first child. By the time I was a rebellious teenager, I was confined to boarding school. There, I enjoyed doing the minimum of work, sang with gusto in the choir, cheated outrageously in maths and latin, but felt at home in geometry and the arts. I never received any special attention from my biological parents, and in return afforded them little thought other than respecting the high learning and expertise of my father in literature, music and painting; a world in which his judgement was prized.

Why had I chosen all these parents? Adding insult to injury, the earliest memories of my grandmother were filled with antipathy. She used to bend over my cot and pinch the bridge of my nose, and rubbing it with olive oil, hiss, 'You look like a Chinese; your eyes are funny and your nose flat. We must do something about it.' I loathed her.

The relationship with my own daughter was of a completely different kind. The moment she was placed on my stomach with head lifted in a bellow backed by the crash of a freak thunderclap and a flash of lightning, I thought of my mother, and was horrified that she could have given away one of her children. Obviously, she had not felt the same immediate bond I had sensed with my daughter with whom I knew there was a deep connection from a previous life. To prove it, memories of a reincarnation long since past crowded into my mind. This had frequently happened to me in childhood. Scenes, incredibly rapid, flicked behind my eyes. I recognised in her the reborn soul I, a childless wife, had loved and nursed to health several hundred years ago in Tibet. Her father, a rich Chinese merchant off with his caravan, had left his young daughter desperately sick in my care, and for a year the joy of her presence had enriched my life until one morning near the end of summer she was taken away crying silently behind the curtains of her canopy perched on a camel bound for her home. The wheel had now turned; she had returned to obliterate the pain in the memory of our parting.

What would the Amchi say if I told him all this? Undoubtedly, nothing short of a sermon on aversion. I opted to keep quiet. But to give credit where credit is due, perhaps I had chosen my real mother for her animal courage, and my handsome father for his beautiful physique. He had style, brains and humour; not such a bad choice in retrospect. I owe them the genetic architecture that shelters my errant soul. Just before my father died, he wrote one of his rare letters asking forgiveness for his rejection. It was easy to forgive him. He had placed me on a path apart, and unwittingly it had proved advantageous in many ways. I would not be here with Sonam were the circumstances of my birth different from what they are. I had escaped into a wider world.

The body, said Sonam, is brought into being by the mixing of seminal fluid and menstrual blood. From the father comes bone, marrow, skin, flesh and blood. The internal organs originate from the mother. Nazir did his best to explain the existence and function of ovules, but the Amchi was not familiar with them and returned to home ground.

'The primal cause of conception, I repeat', he said, 'is Desire. The incarnating one is drawn into existence by attraction to parents whose karma and merits are similar to its own. The Elements gather together and precipitate its form.'

I realised I had better forget about biology, or Sonam's mode of karmic awareness and the choice of parents would become impossibly complicated. One sperm out of myriads squirming their way to the fulfilment of fertilisation, is the first to arrive at the ovum. Our individuality and our sex depend on this apparently random procedure. Every sperm cell holds a different arrangement of genes. Had my conception been the result of a different sperm, I might be similar, but never the same as I am ... which was the aim of my 'desire'. In this light, the Buddhist choice of parents is but the first hurdle in events incompatible with contemporary science.

'How,' I asked, 'could an incarnating consciousness direct the combination of semen and menstrual blood to produce a body's sex?'

Sonam sighed. He pondered before answering. 'We have categories of existing things. They are determined by their characteristics, and we are trained to understand them as objects of knowledge; not as things in themselves, independent of an enquirer.'

The enquirer, in this case, was the incarnating being whose desire-filled consciousness ordered the vagaries of genetic combination. Mind, for Sonam, was the root of all phenomena. At present, we study the behaviour of our physiological entity through progressively abstract techniques. One day, we may come to a fuller understanding of matter as the 'intricate collection or grouping of events' that will dovetail into Sonam's ancient teachings and the consequences of Desire.

Rene Descartes, in his *Treatise on the Passions of the Soul* claimed that because the soul or mind was so immense in its comprehension, it could not possibly be confined to the body, or dominated by the needs of the flesh. He thought of the body as a mechanism controlled by the animal spirits which inhabit it. In modern language, these could be the biochemical secretions and substances that order our physical activity.

The perceptions of the soul were believed to be the cause of emotion and its physical and mechanical expressions. While most people still thought that the soul resided in the heart, Descartes was convinced that its seat lay within the pineal gland. In time, emotions and perceptions became functions embedded in neurophysiology, and were, like memory, located in areas of the brain. The soul, dislodged from both heart and pineal gland, was relegated by medicine to the domain of philosophers and, of late, to particle physics.

Modern physics opens up several possibilities. The reductionist approach in which matter is reduced to its smallest components has proved inadequate and needs modification. No line distinguishes mind from matter. Is mind merely the electrochemical process of the brain or is it some entity that acts upon our grey matter? Science points to something beyond itself. Meanwhile, the unlocated soul–mind remains a perplexing enigma, an ephemeral presence that persists behind consciousness. It is here. It is there. It is everywhere. It is together with, but separate from the flesh.

I asked the inevitable question. 'You speak of the incarnating individual, yet claim that the ego, our sense of self, is an illusion.'

'We do not believe there is any lasting sense of self. The "lha", the life principle or the "wandering soul" that we talked about in the farm house, is like a light indeed. It passes back and forth between one state and another, appearing in our bodies and departing again. My sense of self is a passing illusion, just an appearance coming from mental and family conditions, and from cultural formation. The illusion is confirmed by the three mental poisons and the people who see me.'

Nazir guided the conversation back to conception. Sonam said that the consciousness of the incarnating child is trapped between the male and the female substances. Amalgamated by the Wind Nopa, a thread of life materialises which is sustained and developed through the interaction of the five Elements. Their powers bring forth the network of subtle channels[2] round which the physique takes its form. 'Our knowledge of the embryo's weekly progress is more complete than its Indian source that deals solely with monthly change.' said Sonam. 'From the very start, the child's consciousness is in the embryo and nursed by the Wind Nopa, growth passes through the stages we call the "fish", the "turtle", and the "pig". By the sixth month, the foetus senses pleasure or sadness depending on the mother's emotional state.

'Almost 900 years ago, one of our saint-doctors and philosophers described the child's discomfort in the womb. When the mother overeats, it is like being crushed between stones. If food is too little, it is like being suspended in air. If sex is too violent, it feels as if you are being flagellated by thorns. In the twenty-sixth week, come memories of past lives, usually forgotten at birth unless the baby is a Tulku.'

Tibetan anatomy had advanced beyond its early Ayurvedic origins. At death, the body is either burned, buried, or embalmed if it belonged to a holy man. In Lhasa bodies are still cut up and left for birds of prey; a tradition that has given doctors the chance to follow the paths of nerves, tendons and blood vessels. Notwithstanding, anatomical drawings leave much to be desired. The kidneys have no connection with the formation of urine, which falls into the bladder straight from the intestines. Such details were probably unimportant since internal organs were not mechanisms to be dissected to ascertain their functions, but centres of subtle energy. Bones, on the other hand, were carefully classified into types and their quantity meticulously recorded. Tibetan medicine, as Sonam had underlined, is a medicine of constitution: The five Elements and the three Nopas, the theory of the three Mental Poisons and their psychosomatic inference, the tangible anatomy and the Tantric anatomy of the mystic channels. Healing worked on the three levels of mind, energy and matter.

This web of the subtle and tangible had meaning in a culture where medicine went with prayer and many of the physicians/ saints had been meditative monks. If the subtle energy at the core of yoga discipline is impeded in its circulation, the diminished life force leaves room for sickness. Consequently by practising controlled breathing used, for instance, in Hatha Yoga, the body, filled with prana's subtle energy, repels illness. In practice, methods of opening and clearing the mystic channels by breath, belong more to the monasteries than to the public domain.

Every Tibetan accepts that the visible universe and the human form come into existence only to be reabsorbed into their origin at the end of a cosmic or individual life span. Their philosophy begins with the great invisible that manifests itself down to the tiniest of tangibles. We, on the other hand, take the concrete and reduce it to the infinitely small. Even so, western physics in their research on sub-atomic particles, work on the premise that under or over a certain order of magnitude, such building blocks for matter no longer exist; just a tissue of relationships between the various aspects of the whole.

At death, with the disintegration of the flesh, the three Nopas, messengers of the Elements, depart. The Wind blows back through the universe, the Phlegm returns to coagulate the particles in space, the Bile withdraws into the primal Fire of Life, and at the same time, like a rainbow in autumn, individuality disappears.

'In our texts it is written,' said the Amchi, 'the forces of Earth are absorbed into the Element Water. Form falls apart. The forces of Water are absorbed into Fire. The orifices dry up. The forces of Fire are drawn in Air. The body's heat re-assembles itself.[3] The forces of air are taken into Space. Breathing comes to an end. The incarnating being departs and his constituents are reformed in another existence between earthly lives. The Amchi would have appreciated the words of St John Perse:

> There were great winds on the face of the earth;
> Great joyous winds throughout the world.
> Neither were they confined nor sheltered,
> They left men of chaff in the straw year of their wanderings
> Ah yes! . . . great winds on the face of all that live.

NOTES

[1] In Tibetan medicine, the brain is sometimes seen as the sixth sense and thought as a sensorial function directed by consciousness that flows through the subtle channels. Recent research in the West has shown that biochemical secretions are produced by the brain in response to emotion and sensation.

[2] As a foetus develops, the three nopas, interact with a subtle network of invisible channels. These are called the Channels of Genesis. First, are the Channels of Existence, linked to the development of each of the five senses and the consciousness. Second, are the Channels of Liaison, or the vital channels connected with the formation of blood, the circulatory system, internal organs, the nervous system and the brain. Finally, the Channels of Life accompany the Wind Nopa to support the life principle linked to the soul (see below).

BILE WIND PHLEGM

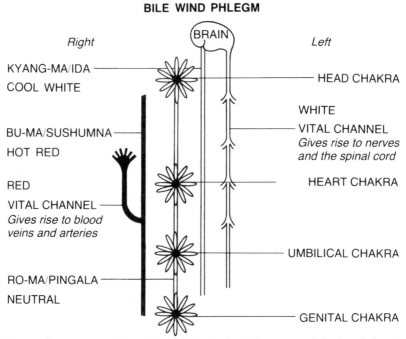

Schematic representation of the subtle body in the areas of the head, heart, umbilical and genital chakras

[3] As heat leaves the body, the metabolism or chemical process of a living cell comes to an end.

FIVE

————————— • —————————

*Our return to a small celebration in camp—A
visit to Sonam's son in the monastery—
Discussions on medicines, the Elixir of Life,
mystic pills, miraculous statues, mantras,
monastic life and the art of making rain*

A SMALL CELEBRATION

A brisk walk with the sun warming our backs took us back to
the village where our horses had been put out to grass. Thelmy
hailed a friend, and the boys ran off singing to catch and saddle
our mounts. By the time we reached the farmhouse, all was ready
for the journey to Karsha. The Amchi's presence, as usual, brought
the people from the fields to wave farewell, and strung with our
belongings, the ponies carried us away in puffs of dust.

We galloped into camp at sunset to find Sonam's friends and
family gathered in a lively reception. From their voices rising into
the heights with repeated cries of 'Julay!' anyone would have
thought it was the return of conquering heroes. The women in
turquoise head-dresses clapped and cheered. The children stood
by with admirable patience until we had taken refreshments, tea
and biscuits handed round by Gulam and Mohamed with an
aplomb that outmatched, by far, their grubby clothes.

It may have been our camp, but the self assurance of the Ladakhis
turned them into our hosts and us their guests. The children sang
an almost perfect rendition of 'Frere Jacques'. Vigorous claps from
audience and performers brought them to their own folk songs,
haunting tunes that floated away through the silence, free from
the bodies that expressed them. The very air, the medium of their
existence, linked the sounds and their creators to the heavens above
the bastion of mountains protecting us from the outside world.

Sonam asked us to dance. Nazir and I composed ourselves, and solemnly singing the 'Blue Danube', we waltzed round and round to collapse, lungs bursting, at his feet.

'That was a good!' said Nazir in a pant.

'Yes,' replied Sonam with a slow nod. 'All experiences are a form of medicine. They resemble ingredients gathered from many places. Some are sweet, others bitter, and they wait to be purified into a draught of wisdom. Now, we will sleep. Tomorrow, we go to the monastery. My youngest son, Pema, has his cell filled with herbs and you will learn more about remedies.'

MEMORIES

In the small hours of a restless night, I mulled over Sonam's remarks, and realised that for him, medicine, inseparable from his faith, was much more than the art of healing. It was the art of living itself. How many lives had I lived since birth? An African childhood interrupted at the age of three with two years in London; balloons held by a fat lady at the gates of Hyde Park; a white fur coat, red shoes, street lamps in the fog outside the nursery window. From England, I sailed home to grow up on pewter sands by seas crashing against the shores of the Cape of Good Hope. In clear memory I drifted into the hinterland of vines beside oak forests and white gabled homesteads built by my ancestors, the Huguenots. In memory I passed on to desert farms and the savannas, yellow in winter grass, falling into the heat of the bushveldt. At seventeen, I left the Cape, so beautiful, so smug in its suburban luxury, for student days in London. A call from my family took me back to southern sunshine, a brief first marriage and a nine month-old son. Two fragile beings, we were towed by the currents of my restlessness across Europe until our lives were given security in a second marriage. As the Amchi had said, I had gathered precious ingredients from distant places, but I had not, as yet, compounded them into an elixir. Much healing had still to be done, and before dawn, pictures of dancing swung through my mind.

Snow flutters down quiet as white moths. The big flakes swirl about and settle, glistening, in front of the floodlit facade of Schonbrun, in Vienna. I waltz tirelessly, and in a kaleidoscope of colour merged with sound, figures caught by the candlelight move across gilt and glass. The reflections are given life by the music as they whirl in their glittering world of mirrors. That evening, love is a magic mirror that protects me from everyday reality. Secreted away in my memory, in lone moments I review the scene with a miser's meanness lest it be tarnished by an intruder. In the Zangskar, for the first time my memories hold no pain.

VISIT TO KARSHA

The next day bloomed from behind the mountains. In the early morning air free of dust, details in the landscape had a vividness and the hallucinating quality of dreams experienced in high fever. During breakfast, we watched the ferrymen paddle a pair of hardkneed hikers across the river. A gaggle of children stood on our side of the bank to welcome them with the best of Gallic gestures reserved for wordless insults picked up from travellers. The hikers were at first confused and then amused.

'Those were not exactly signs of international friendship,' I grunted to Nazir, 'what happens if the kids do that to the monks?'

'A sound whack on the backside with a heavy stick will be what they get. The monks get around and are not as isolated as one might think.'

A light chuckle came from behind. The Amchi stood over us in his soft, leather boots. Arriving unheard, he was ready to leave for Karsha, where his son, Pema was preparing to take his place amongst the 160 monks at the fifteenth century monastery.

Our gradual ascent turned into a hard climb. Monks streaked up and down past us, always with a greeting, black boots flashing out from maroon robes held up in their hands. They made me feel uncouth, a sick goat in the noonday heat, plodding on, quite breathless. Sonam, having gone ahead, stood with Pema just below the monastery on the roof of a small white house. They waved, but in the maze of paths, Nazir and I missed the entrance, climbed too high, and with some well chosen curses, panted our way down again.

In the final climb to Pema's room by an almost perpendicular stairway cut in the rock, we entered and sighed at the view. Perched high above the valley, I looked out, longing to fly with the eagles that glided and swooped and hovered over the land below. Earthbound, I slumped to the floor. The scent of dried herbs came from his bed covered with plants. A table, chair, one worn sheepskin, robes on a peg and the inevitable magazine pictures of the Dalai Lama were all Pema's worldly possessions. Between study and prayer, he worked as a tailor making and repairing clothes for his colleagues. Otherwise, life in the monastery only gave time off for family visits and collecting herbs in the mountains with his father.

TIBETAN MEDICINES AND THE ELIXIR OF LIFE

Traditionally, an apprentice identifies plants by sight, smell and taste. Later, blindfolded, he will be expected to recognise anything up to 200 among the 2200 entered in the texts. Formulas contain up to seventy-five ingredients prepared in pills and powders, or as pastes, herbal teas and oils. Bark is collected in spring, flowers, fruit and seeds in summer and autumn, leaves and resin in late summer, roots, stems and branches before winter sets in. Every part of a plant has its use: roots for the bones and to clear the channels, stems for the flesh, leaves for the internal organs, flowers acted on the senses and fruit is good for the heart and also the internal organs. 'Our analogy between the body and the plant comes from the attraction between things of a similar nature,' said Sonam.

Extracts from vegetable and micro-organisms make up well over half of our Western pharmacopoeia, but the profit motive in research makes it difficult to collect material in the remote Himalayas. Indiscriminate prescription of antibiotics had led to increased resistance of bacteria. Soon 80–90 per cent of all germs will be immune to their action, thus any substance helping the immune system is of value. I told Sonam that our chemists analyse traditional compounds, isolate the active ingredients and reproduce them synthetically. However, since a traditional medicine consists of diverse compounds and never a sole component, isolated constituents often lack the physiological effect of the original organic mixture. The ancients knew, within limits, what was involved in chemical reaction. For example, it was forbidden to cut the roots of the ginseng plant with anything but a bamboo knife. Modern research shows why. If iron comes into contact with ginseng's anti-ageing agent, maltol, it destroys the antioxidant properties which guard against cellular deterioration.

Another discovery from China is a pain killer for cancer taken from the secretions of toads' taste buds, and added to herbal components, this has a 92 per cent success rate with no toxic side effects.

Sonam listened; Nazir translated making sure the Amchi realised the cost involved in research. He threw back his head in laughter. I was always amazed how he kept his hat on during his gusts of hilarity.

'We don't have those problems here, although price is involved when a precious ingredient is needed. Sometimes jewels and gold and silver are taken from the monastery's treasure. They have to be purified before we mix them with other things.'

A base of turquoise, red or blue, is used for lung and liver infections. There are usually two grades of precious medicines. Pearls, the best tinged with red, act on the brain and absorb poisons. Oyster shells and mother of pearl are the second choice just as sapphire quartz flecked with gold is inferior to the plain kind. Both are found in compounds for leprosy and to counteract poisons. Gold is also used to combat poison. Beaten thin as a fly's wing, it is cut and ground, then pounded into power with brimstone, black sesame, linum (flower, stem and leaves) rock salt, borax and water. Rolled into small balls, it is put into an iron pot, sealed and left over a fire until the mixture is reduced to ash. For centuries, syphillis has been treated with mercury compounds. White lead relieves certain skin afflictions, iron, brass, copper and tin also have their merits. Lapis regulates the fluids, coral reduces high blood pressure, malachite soothes the nerves.

One formula, based on purified mercury, is called 'The Elixir of Life'. In mythical times, two gods churned the ocean for this elixir but a huge, black serpent surged up and spread its poison into life on earth. Eight powers ate the beast and a king emerged to reign in terror. His name was Mercury. Eight wise men knew the secret of turning the king into a magic potion. To do so they first had to get him drunk. The queen, a fickle woman, decided to help. Using her wiles, he was bound and transformed. The queen's name was Sulphur.

In 1980, the Dalai Lama with the help of the Indian Government, obtained the release from Lhasa of a famous Tibetan doctor, Tensing Choedrak. He had survived seventeen years of imprisonment with hard labour, and was said to be the only person alive who knew the secret of making the elixir. In Daramsala, distillation began on a day carefully chosen by astrologers, the 28th of March, 1982.

After all due prayer and rites, the process of getting Mercury drunk began. The liquid metal was first rolled and kneaded with spices in the heat resistant skins of the rare Musk deer. As work progressed, the men drank a mixture of chang and urine to counter-act the toxic fumes. After four days, the mercury no longer separated into small pellets. The final consistency was found when match sticks remained upright in the coagulated mass. Plastic bags were then put over the skin containers. Ingredients included sulphur, gold, gold ore, copper, tin, iron fillings, various mineral rocks, and a wide range of plant and animal substances. It took one and a half months to prepare the mixture; each metal was purified, covered with a paste, wrapped in white cloth and dried in the sun. Gold, after similar treatment, was baked in crucibles in an open kiln tended day and night. The end result, taken as a powder or a pill, has been used to boost similarly prepared medicines based on the purification of precious stones. These secret recipes, often passed on from one medical Lama to another, are reserved for acute conditions requiring formulas of exceptional potency. Patients tended by Lamas in America and Europe claim they have had relief from pain in liver and kidney disorders, remission and even cures from some forms of cancer in its early stages.

'All Nature's products have a medicinal use,' said Sonam. 'Everything from excreta to jewels, and I make poultices of hot pigeon dung for boils. We classify medicines and food by taste. Taste comes from the materialised essence of the five Elements. Six flavours arise from their intermingling. Earth and Water products have a sweet taste. Fire and Water, salty, and so forth. Sweet, acid, salty and spicy tastes battle against the disturbed Wind Nopa. Bitter and astringent tastes rectify the Bile. Sour and salty flavours react on the Phlegm.

'I first judge a formula's action by taste which indicates the potential "hot" or "cold" energy that will be released after digestion. As some tastes change in digestion, I must estimate the effects if the basic substance is mixed with others since the final result will differ from its theoretical flavour.'

This relationship between taste and Element came from Indian oral tradition which associated the physical effects of certain plants with their flavour. Into this system came the Chinese and Græco-Arab concept of medicines and food being either 'hot' or 'cold' in their potency and in their effects. Where these two systems failed to blend in practice, they were integrated by the idea of postdigestive change releasing an energy that differed from its theoretical source.

In this way, theory married abstract speculation to empirical observations. The power Sonam spoke of was the principle that all things of the same category energise each other while those of an opposite nature pacify. Formulas of a Fire Element regulate the cool Phlegm Nopa. Plants of a Water nature calm the hot Bile Nopa. The Wind Nopa, basically neutral, becomes either hot or cold depending on its imbalance.

Neat and ingenious, these theories endow our common material with arcane significance. The Buddhists' sophisticated speculations were the mature extensions of man's primal identification with an environment to whose powers he submitted himself and the contents of his world. Nature and the human body alike, had been formulated in terms of mystical concentrations of energy that gave both poetic meaning and practical significance to the day-by-day trials and errors of scholarly physicians.

DIAGNOSTICS, DEATH AND DEVOTION

One Summer, I had spent a week on the island of Madura in Indonesia with a 'Dukun'. Ambiguous figures, they can be mediums and necromancers as well as herbalists and healers. Women of the island are prized for the muscular contractions executed in a sexual proficiency assured to leave their men in a state of considerable satisfaction. In the month after childbirth, a stretched birth passage is fast restored to tautness with preparations from, among other things, barks, herbs, seeds, dried fruit and fungi. The old Dukun I visited took pride in her remedies. Outwardly an orthodox Moslem, like most Indonesians, she kept faith with the supernatural. She insisted that all her knowledge came from her grandmother's instructions heard in dreams she had had since her fourteenth year. I did not entirely believe her. The basic products were commonly known, and varied only in proportions and mixtures which the Dukun consulted. However, I had witnessed Zulu Sangoma (women or homosexual mediums who contact ancestral spirits) in full trance diagnose and prescribe medicines showing uncanny precision in predicting where they could be freshly procured. I readily accepted the seed of truth in the Dukun's chaff. Extra-sensory perception can, in one form or another, play a part in the selection of opportune ingredients. But the Dukun and the Sangoma were passive receivers. Sonam, and any first class Amchi, if wishing to experiment with his own formulas, apply an intuition heightened by meditation, and gathering their wits, actively use them.

Diagnosis begins with a set of twenty questions, followed by pulse and urine analysis and a physical examination. A yellow coated, furry tongue indicates a disturbed Bile Nopa, a rough, dry tongue an upset Wind Nopa, and a white coating, an unsettled Phlegm. Stage by stage the Amchi decides on the attitude he will adopt for a cure.

'Sometimes' said Sonam, 'If my diagnosis is uncertain, I heal the way a cat stalks a mouse. Should I be dealing with an unresponsive disease, I act like somebody steering a team of horses along a chosen route. To avoid side effects in cases when all three Nopas are disturbed, I am a chief settling quarrels. I judge the various side effects of a medicine by examining stools, urine and sweat. The intensity of my therapy will depend on the season, the state and age of the patient and the location of his complaint. The most basic treatments pacify the Nopas. If they are not successful, I use emetics from Fire and Earth plants for disorders on the upper part of the body and purgatives from Water and Earth plants for the lower areas.'

'What happens, honoured Amchi, if treatment fails and you know the patient is going to die?'

'We do our best. Death is a more important time and can be frightening if you are not ready for the physical sensations as the body breaks down. A priest recites prayers to help open the crown chakra for the consciousness to leave the flesh. Complete release from the body is hastened by returning it to the Elements. It can be burnt if wood is not scarce, thrown into water . . . a common funeral for children under a year-old . . . or dismembered, the bones and flesh pounded up with blessed barley paste and left for the vultures. The carnal envelope is given back to the Air. Burial is rare and not honourable. The Earth belongs to the lower entities.'

'But if a person is in great pain, do you help him die more peacefully with medicines to dull the suffering?'

The Amchi shook his head. 'The Lamas don't approve. Medicines that dull pain also affect the mind. And in the Bardo, the intermediary state between lives, it is better to have an alert and unconfused consciousness, otherwise the terrifying phantoms projected from your mind will hinder and prevent you from being attracted to a good reincarnation. We help the consciousness from the moment it leaves the body. At first, it hovers for three or four days, barely separated from the corpse before being drawn into the Bardo for forty-nine days where it prepares itself for a future existence.

'If the consciousness leaves by the head chakra, depending on karma, the next life can be in the realm of gods, demi-gods or humans. If it departs through the lower orifices, rebirth occurs in the form of a demon or animal. We have a supply of special pills, mystic pills given with the blessing of great Lamas, sometimes even the Dalai Lama. They carry a spiritual force and emit the light of the life principle transferred into them by saintly men, and in some cases, pieces of their bones, fingernails or hair which carry the aura of their spiritual power.'

These relics, carried in amulets, also bestow protection against wounds and sickness. Some pills are said to multiply spontaneously although they are made only from roasted grain mixed with scented water. The paste is rolled into balls coated with red dye. The Abbot, shaven headed and appropriately robed, puts the pills into a perfectly formed jar, which, when two thirds full, is wrapped, tied and left in an upright position. A 'dorje', emblem of the thunderbolt, is wrapped and fastened to the jar's neck to add its vibrations for the hundred-day alchemical ritual. Invocations continue without a break, repeated by relays of monks fed on wheat cakes and buttered tea during the ceremonies. Unlike other times, they pay strict attention to their personal cleanliness. At the end of each day, the dorje, or an idol on top of the vase, is washed before the room is perfumed with burning sandalwood or twigs of juniper.

The notion of Tantric rituals of ablution took me back to India's richest temple at Tirumalai where thousands of pilgrims arrive to worship the statue of Venkateswara. Venerated for his power in answering prayers and inducing miraculous cures, he is a magnet for all Hindu sects. They worship Venkateswara not as an idol but as a manifestation of Vishnu, the Preserver. A manifestation implies that an object is permeated by the deity's awareness, whereas an incarnation is the god's self-chosen presence in a living body. Escorted through outer halls and along a passage into the womb-like room of the inner sanctum, I stood breathless from the magnificence of the scene. The nine-foot high statue of black stone was ablaze with jewels. Venkateswara's head bore a beehive crown of gold massed with precious stones, and beneath it, curved a white mask of purified camphor to shield his eyes and leave judgement to his inner sight. Chains of twenty-two carat gold hung from his shoulders, one weighing seventy pounds bore enormous links studded with diamonds. The diamond-encrusted epaulettes, gauntlets and leg shields scintillated under torchlight illuminating other enamelled ornaments set with sapphires and rubies. A great emerald, three and a half inches wide, glowed on his chest. As priests circled with torches, white fire leapt from a myriad of gems. Gold statues, his consorts, glittered next to gold receptacles on the floor.

The head priest was a physiologist trained at Stanford University in America. 'Often when I bathe the Lord, and anoint his chest,' he confided, 'there seems to be a living vibration emanating from his body, and when I run my hands over the stone, I feel every muscle and sinew as if it were alive. I don't know what kind of stone it is, but the camphor mask, which is usually corrosive, has left no mark even after over 1300 years of recorded rites.' A few days later, the impact was no less intense. This time, the god was adorned with beauty of a different order. Garlands upon garlands of flowers covered his form.

The aura of sanctity and the allure of splendour, mysticism and materialism has kept this temple famous and immensely rich with donations from thankful devotees. One old Brahmin official commented with infuriating self-satisfaction; 'The Buddha is just another form of Vishnu, and from our Vedic philosophy came Tantric Buddhism, its symbols and practices rearranged to suit Tibetan Lamaism. Buddhism? It should be labelled "Hinduism for export only".' 'I quite agree,' I said. 'One's best products should always be kept for export.'

MONASTIC LIFE

Three young monks came into Pema's room. He rose from the herb-covered bed. It was time for prayers. Time for gongs and drums and deep chants; a sound that hit the pit of the stomach to rise and fill the head with the noise of a celestial beehive. The drums' deep thwacks and the long horns booming resembled the groans from a bull tethered underground. Sounds of the earth itself. The winds sweeping through the valley were echoed in the wail of trumpets and conch shells, cacophonous voices of nature often far from pleasant to western ears.

Certain prayers are accompanied by such music. Those marked by bells and rattles are chanted on two notes. Those incanted to the sound of cornets and other instruments, waver between four notes and an octave.

Pema was preparing himself to take his place among the 160 monks in Karsha monastery with its 239 acres of land and thirteen villages with a further thirteen attached by religious affiliation to the reformed Gelugpa order headed by the Dalai Lama.

'Why have you left so many of your mantras written in sanskrit?' asked Nazir.

'We pronounce "seed syllables", and believe they carry the power of sound that would be lost if translated,' replied the Amchi. 'We recite them at different volumes. Some are chanted, others whispered or hummed. They guard against seasonal illness, epidemics, or are pronounced to arouse the chakras. Different schools have different methods. Other mantras are used like a general pill for health and some include visualisation of a particular aspect of the Buddha to invoke his blessings in healing. But I am a country doctor, not an ordained priest.'

In the Vedic doctrine, long before the Buddha, all form is fashioned by sound, the soul of shape. Behind any thought rests an unheard vibration. The first manifestation of sound was light – luminous sound – and from this point spread lines that crystallised into ideas and matter. Everything has its particular density of vibration. Seers, adepts in mantras or thought forms strung symbolic syllables together which resonate in the subtle body. The mysteries of the mantra were mastered by a few and passed on to a very small number of initiates. Today, the masses drone to subdue their minds, and at the incredible speed at which mantras are recited, meaning falls into their subconscious. On another level, continued Sonam, mantra vibrations, repeated over the centuries, have left reverberations like a path in Space; a road to virtue. There is nothing devotional in a mantra. It is not prayer, but a mystical formula that invokes the permanent power of sound in the process of continual transition.

'I agree with the idea behind all this,' said Nazir. 'We know that sound shatters glass and if certain vibrations are passed through a thin metal sheet covered with sand, the sand takes on a pattern. But, to what degree a mantra can alter the body's workings, I leave open to question.'

Why, we asked Sonam, if the monks prayed and recited with perpetual fervour, were they also prone to illness? 'It could be from a distant cause in karma,' said Sonam, 'or present circumstance as well. They are compassionate and vulnerable, and take on themselves the poison of others.' Pema, who had waited for the end of the conversation, shook hands. Time to go. Sonam had his own business. He promised to see us soon. 'I will then have a surprise for you.' He turned and preceded us down the stairs, and our ways parted outside the house. My knees ached as we clambered down hill. 'Ladakh, land of the leaping Lamas.' I rolled the alliteration off my tongue at the spectacle of monks springing upwards towards us. 'Lama is the Tibetan word for guru, and means 'the superior one', said Nazir.

Only two classes of monks have the right to be called Lama. The first are Tulkus, usually from the noble class, exceptions proving the rule. They are reincarnations of highly respected Lamas, often heads of monasteries, and sometimes their past lives can be traced back to the gurus of India who first brought Buddhism to the North, or established and reformed the creed after it had arrived in Tibet. Others can trace their lives back to the Buddha's disciples. This was the case with Kushok Bakula, the spiritual leader of Ladakh and representative of the Gelugpa sect.

Astrologers and oracles predict the birth of Tulkus, especially the Dalai and Panchen Lama. If a child prattles about memories of a past life in a particular monastery, he is taken there to be judged by the Lamas who knew him, and tested to see if he recognises ritual objects, possessions and friends. If all is well, he is accepted and given intensive training with privileges that go far beyond those normal for his age. Tulkus learn the Dharma by heart, and when grown to manhood receive special Tantric disciplines and oral transmissions. The Guru-Lama of a Tulku is given the deepest respect. Oral instruction includes receiving the spiritual power of the teacher. Not every guru can directly pass this blessing to his pupil. Parents have been known to refuse their Tulku child entrance into the monastery, preferring him to have a normal, less rigorous education for a job or profession. Such cases are rare, and should this happen, the life of a Tulku usually comes to an abrupt end; some outside force causes untimely death.

They can't all be Tulkus, and Pema is a tailor, I reflected as another group of monks passed us.

The saffron robes prescribed by the Buddha were unsuitable for the North, and since the northern school of Buddhism is noted for its inclination to follow the spirit rather than the letter of the law, the dress was soon modified. A monk's skirt is made of eight yards of material sewn in to rectangular patches in tribute to the rags of holy men. Pleats on the left and right hip face different directions depending on whether the wearer is a follower of the Dalai or Panchen Lama. The number of pleats vary with the sects. Sometimes the upper toga has a front and back panel of Chinese brocade, a fashion originating from the twelfth Dalai Lama's mother when she spent all her money on a beautiful piece of material stitched onto her son's garment. The dimensions of the outer robe are measured according to the monk's purse. Worn over the left shoulder and under the right arm, its colour depends on the local dye. In Tibet, a terracota red takes the place of Ladakh's more magenta hue. An extra garment commonly worn today, is a sleeveless yellow or red cotton shirt. The standard Gelugpa cap of mustard felt rises to a point and has wide flaps turned up over the ears to show a red lining.

Nazir, with a descriptive flourish of his hands, said that the yellow head-dress with crest like a horse's mane, and worn in processions, originated from the soldiers of Alexander the Great. 'They were taken over by the Shamans and later grabbed by the Buddhists who knew a spectacular decoration when they saw one.'

No monk owns more than his clothes, prayer books, writing table, tea kettle, cups and, hopefully, a wool or sheepskin rug. Money is handed out for razors and writing materials. The monastic official responsible for finances, buys oil for lamps, tea and provisions, and sells the produce from the monastery's lands: grain, fruit, wood, yak, sheep and goats.

'They write either in the sacred script or in a running hand,' said Nazir. 'A number of monks I have come across only know how to count on their fingers, and many Tibetan ideas on science are pre-Copernician.'

Contact with the West, I remarked, must have left some trace. The monk were surely more advanced now than in 1904 when the British military mission marched into Tibet. On that occasion, a certain Abbot, when informed that the earth was round, instructed the Europeans, with courteous condescension and a singular lack of interest, to read better books. Half the world was shaped like a shoulder of mutton and contained Tibet, he had said.

Nazir smiled and shook his head. 'You know another strange thing. Many of the monks may be interested in science and technology and radios and jeeps. But in some monasteries they hold the secret of making rain'. I wanted him to be more specific. 'Well!' he gave a cough, 'in Rizong, a place way over there in the northwest, forty years ago, a British commission dashed off to verify the claim and ended up by declaring it was valid but quite inexplicable.' Nazir had often been there, a world apart lying below its massive peaks.

'What did you find out?' I asked, noting the distant look in his eyes. He stopped. We had passed onto open ground, and he crouched down to light a cigarette.

THE ART OF MAKING RAIN

'I asked them if it was true that they could make rain. Yes, they said, How? I asked, and they told me they went off into the mountains and chanted from texts for a couple of days. What texts? I asked. Were they to do with the climate? They laughed and said No, not the way you might think. Each monk takes a leaf from a book and repeating it at his own rate, he mumbles away at top speed. After a few hours of this, by evening, rain falls. Simple! What happens if they overdo it and floods arrive? They have one set of manuscripts for making rain and another for stopping it. They just told me the texts came from a treaty called "The Elixir of Life", like the mercury medicine. What's more, they said that the monastery had lost half the pages!'

Before the Dalai Lama fled his homeland, he ordered many copies to be made of the sacred books, the hundred volumes of the scriptures and the two hundred others of commentary. They wrapped them all in cloth and transported the loads on the monk's backs across the Himalayas into India. 'Dharma, the laws to overcome Karma and reach Nirvana,' muttered Nazir. 'They say, destroy the Dharma and the Dharma destroys you. Sonam knows a lot, yet he never seems to be burdened by it all. Perhaps he too, like Choedrak, has received oral secrets from his guru.'

'If he has, they are for his and not our ears!'

The Amchi had studied long. He continued to learn, test and observe, and with his keen intelligence most likely had devised some of his own remedies marked in his notebook. The taxing climate and physical conditions in the Zangskar had furrowed his brow and lined his cheeks. He had lost his wife. But even so, no inner scars veiled his eyes. Each day, they sparkled as he looked at life's events. He, who denied any permanence of the self, with his modesty and humour, had a remarkable density to his being, a residual core, as strong and durable as the rocks around us. He had said he would return soon. When, was an unnecessary question.

SIX

•

Tantric sex—The story of Tibet's most famous woman doctor—Evil spirits, possessions, Shamans, and religious festivals

TANTRIC SEX AND MONASTIC LIFE

The wind blew with an aggravating whine. It drove us into the mess tent with its heavy aroma of food. Even the shepherd children had abandoned their goats for cover behind hillocks. Today, no passing visits came from friendly monks on their way down to Padum for provisions, or, as one of them liked to say in carefully pronounced English, 'Important buzz-iness', an importance never divulged most likely through lack of vocabulary.

That morning, Nazir, seldom at a loss for a good yarn, entertained me with anecdotes from his visits to the different monasteries. 'Only one of the four main orders are authorised to marry,' he said, 'and the monks, I can tell you, are often far from saintly. They're a randy bunch and not averse to their own kind.'

Buddhists have an ambivalent approach to sex and the body. Influenced by Tantrism and Hindu alchemy, sulphur and mercury had been used from the seventh century in an effort to attain eternal youth ... a far cry from the early disciples, who, intent on an escape from time and suffering, emphasised a doctrine of renunciation. Desire, the cause of procreation, had to be tamed by celibacy. Paradoxically, dogma could not deny the right for a human being to be born. Experience in this world had value, and truth had to be seen in its absolute as well as its relative context.

In some monasteries, following the teachings of Tantric yoga, monks strove to transmute sexual energy and direct it into the subtle channels with their junctions in the chakras. Sexual organs were symbols to be read on different levels. The ritual objects of the 'Thunderbolt' (phallus) and the 'Lotus' (vagina), held a spiritual or carnal connotation depending on the circumstances. Union between the active, and receptive principles could be an entirely mental process affecting the mystic body, or it could be realised in participation with a female partner. Initiates knew the effect of rhythmic mantras incanted to stimulate the chakras, and by mastering the muscles that acted on the neurovascular system and the endocrine secretions in the pelvic area, they avoided what was considered as a loss of vitality and psychic energy in orgasm. Semen, they believed, only collected itself in one area during climax, otherwise, 'like the juice in sugar cane' it was an essence of the vital force carried throughout the body.

Since we all have within us both masculine and feminine qualities, meditation, grounded in *coitus reservatus*, the act of preventing ejaculation by mental control, awoke in man his feminine aspect for a spiritual marriage of his two-fold nature. An actual or an imagined image of a goddess invoked the feminine energy, and in the marriage of his male and female polarities, his retained semen was transmuted into a purified essence permeated by the forces of the five Elements. It was an analogy to marriage and the formation of the embryo that comes into being through the intervention of the cosmic Elements at the moment of conception. The power from the transmuted semen rested in the lowest chakra situated in the genital area from where it was drawn upwards along the subtle channels into the six others, and once opened, like petals of a flower, they glowed with colours beheld by the inner eye. If this exercise, not without danger, was accomplished, the adept lost himself in a state beyond polarity where differentiation no longer exists. Male and female, good and evil, matter and spirit, beginning and end were seen as one.

Sexual mysticism has its parallel in psychology in that the libido, Freud's sexual drive or Jung's vital energy, can be expanded from individual consciousness to embrace the collective. Tantric practice seeks a similar goal by gradually leading the initiate's consciousness into the Chakra's inner realms. These realms, each governed by their own deity are unlocked by meditation and mental direction of subtle energy from the transmuted semen. At first, it is a journey into the dark side of the subconscious where apparitions of fear, repression and violence take the form of demons and gods who can derange an uncontrolled mind. After long training, the initiate guides his energy from the lowest Chakra to the highest one at the crown of the head. If successful, he becomes an adept, and having survived the power of both demons and gods, experiences ultimate awareness.

By the eighth century, when Tibet's contact with China was growing, Buddhism became influenced by Taoist sexual alchemy for physical immortality. Both doctrines shared the concepts of harmonising opposite yet complementary forces, and conserving semen. Coitus reservatus that previously served a mystic end, was turned into a method of transforming the body within time. The goal was not to escape the flesh, but to preserve it with an elixir derived from the sexual act. The man withheld his fluid while absorbing the woman's secretions, and should he release semen, it was sucked back into his system by the muscular control of his urethra. Certain sects even advised that menstrual blood had sedative and regenerative properties.[1]

Prostitutes existed although they were never an organised section of Tibetan society as in ancient China. But by the ninth and tenth centuries, orgies were rife in the monasteries to the point that one king, a monk, wrote indignant criticism of the clergy's degenerate behaviour. Many had embarked on the left hand path of Tantric sex. They ate meat and drank alcohol before mass copulations in which the satisfaction of the grossest instincts replaced the rigours of mysticism.

'All this,' commented Nazir, 'reminds me of an Indian friend I once trekked with. He was a strong fellow, walked well, did hatha yoga and at one time had gone in for Tantric sex. After a couple of years, he decided it was unnatural and didn't like some of the rituals. On occasions, they had an enormously fat woman who became possessed by a goddess. She foamed at the mouth and writhed about with the men jumping on her, each convinced he was screwing the demon-goddess herself.

'More normal sex took place in a room lit with oil lamps, and the mixed group repeated mantras. When the man entered his partner, the guru put a lamp near their private parts. Evidently, the red spectrum excites the man's glands and the violet does the same for the woman. Only the women were allowed their climaxes, so my friend got fed up with this rather one sided affair and wanted his release too. The guru said no. So, after months of frustration and no special advantages other than learning how to keep his erection for a long time, he gave it all up and now pleases the ladies as much as himself. Well, let's get back to the Tibetans. They use aphrodisiacs like bear bile, but I haven't found them obsessed with sex. They discuss it openly and just love ribald jokes.

Luckily, they have escaped the repression of Islam, the prudery of India, and China's puritanism. But, my God! Save me from being one of those Tantric monks overcoming my sexual urges by sitting cross-legged and lighting up my chakras like a bloody Christmas tree!'

Tibetan medicine has much to say about homosexuality. The sexual organs of men and women each possess their energy fields, and in union, the fields harmonise. Mating with the same sex disrupts the normal frequencies and perturbs the mental and physical system. In consequence, the physical imbalance in the hormones produces an emotional distortion supported by behavioural patterns. Homosexuals of both sexes take pills (of animal and vegetable origin) for one week a month. They act on the hormonal system, and the length of treatment depends on the depth of the disturbance.

A FAMOUS WOMAN DOCTOR

I once had interviewed a young woman, Tsewang Dolma, who was the head of the Tibetan clinic in Delhi. Her mother, Lobsang, is one of Tibet's leading doctors, and I told Nazir their story. The daughter is the fourteenth in an unbroken line of family physicians since 1046 when an Indian Tantric master passed through their district in South Tibet. He predicted that 200 years later, they would found a small hospital on the mountain of Khanga, a centre of free healing that would be run by Tsewang's ancestors. Another prophecy foretold a break in the lineage of medicine passed from father to son that would herald dark days for Tibet. Lobsang's birth fulfilled this prediction. She became the first woman Amchi to carry on her family tradition. She graduated from Lhasa in 1958. That same year, she left Tibet with her two daughters strapped on her back. The three of them escaped the Chinese by walking for five days across the Himalayas into Nepal. Amchi Dolma worked as a day labourer on the roads for a year before she had the chance to cure three well known Indians. This brought her recognition, and later, under the patronage of the Dalai Lama, she accepted the position of chief physician in the hospital at Daramsala. By the mid 70s, 20 per cent of her patients came from the West. In due course, Lobsang Dolma trained her daughter to take over the Delhi clinic.

Pretty in a pink sleeveless dress, Tsewang sat in her office under a tanka of the Buddha of Medicine gazing down on the ever-renewed cycles of birth and decay, sickness and health. She cared for epileptics and diabetics, tended children and adults with terrible skin infections, treated the obese, infertile or impotent. The clinic also had its share of terminal cancer cases rejected by the hospitals. 'Beyond the body's malfunctions lie the supernatural, and evil spirits.' she commented 'Our treatment alleviates the symptoms, but in severe cases, unless the patient goes to a Lama for ritual and prayer, the disease returns.' One person in fifty will fall ill through demonic intervention.

Nazir interrupted me saying, 'I'm pretty sure she kept no records to arrive at that percentage. It's the same old story, lots of quality and no verifiable quantity.'

'If the Tibetans believe in exorcism, so does the Catholic Church.' I said.

A DISCUSSION ON EXORCISM

I told Nazir about Father Dominique who lived in a farmhouse in Normandy. After three decades of work in India and Ceylon, this stout and elderly priest had been recalled to France and appointed exorcist of the Paris area. I had seen him in one of his formidable rages, a cold fury that reduced a thick headed, obstinate farmer to a state of shock. The Father was a match for any man and any intruding devil. In his study, awash with papers and piles of obscure books, hung an eight-inch iron crucifix bent by a child of seven. She had attacked him and wrenched the cross from his hands to twist it during exorcism. He freed her. I had asked him why, if the devil and his gang are so powerful, they can't take over anyone of their choice. There must be an inherent disturbance in the person's psyche, he had replied, or possession cannot take place. Ninety-nine per cent of the men, women and children he counselled needed a psychiatrist and not an exorcist. Notwithstanding, Father Dominique recognised the presence of personified evil, as did the Tibetans.

Prior to the arrival of Buddhism, the clans had little more than ritual, sacrifice, effigies and spirit-traps to combat sickness. Spirits entered animals and humans, or took their place on a person's shoulder or head. Should a protective deity leave due to a stain on an individual's character, the 'abandoned one' became prey for evil entities. Father Dominique agreed with the similarity between the Shaman's idea of a stained character and his own conclusion that an inherent psychic flaw could open the door to possession.

As Buddhism gradually spread through Tibet, the Shaman's established belief that spirits could be the cause of illness, was absorbed into the more logical theories of Indian Ayurvedic medicine. Signs of possession were rationalised and coded for diagnosis through pulse and urine analysis. Ancient practices joined to the new reassured a traditional people unwilling to reject the Shaman's hold.

Shamans acted as go-betweens from the human to the spirit world. In their evolution from the neolithic and bronze ages, they were remnants of the food-gathering and hunting stage of man's development when their mediumship brought them to positions of power. Respected and feared, they became clan leaders, chief warriors and even tribal princes. The two categories of Tibetan Shamans were the 'Shen', men and women diviners who did not connect demons to sickness, and the 'Bön', adepts at therapeutic exorcism.

In Ladakh, indigenous beliefs were preserved by the once powerful Bön, advisers to kings, bards and protectors of individuals and society. Not priests of any defined religion, their rites synthesised Chinese Taoism and the Kashmiri cult of worshipping half-human half-serpent water deities. Mythological heroes, through exceptional force and cleverness, interceded between gods and demons for human benefit. Later, the old nature spirits were taken into the Buddhist cosmic landscape, and the Bön's divination and exorcism of destructive entities lived on in the rituals of the educated Lama Exorcists; psychologists in their own right. It left the village Shaman and his self-induced trances on a lower level than the highly trained Amchi, whose knowledge of human behaviour and psychosis went further than common superstition.

The mind is a mirror. Its mental poisons reflect nefarious powers embodied in the evil spirits of the cosmic, terrestrial and lower spheres. Mental therapy in prayer and ritual modifies behaviour, and a concerned and close relationship with the distressed patient aids the work of auto-suggestion. No mentally disturbed person is ever isolated from society for it increases their deranged perceptions. The brain is not a separate organ that can be drugged to suppress symptoms of a deluded consciousness. Such a notion shocks Tibetans since the basic cause of Ignorance lies dormant, waiting to be revived in the future with greater consequences.

SHAMANS

The wind blew on. It hissed outside the tent like a demented demon. In its implacable and mindless search for an entrance, it battered the canvas as if it were our skin that barred its intrusion into our beings. I imagined ancient tribes, wild eyes peering into the mists populated with spirits more numerous than there were men. Fear pulsated around them, seeping into thoughts ravaged by phantoms. As we sat there, scenes of Shamans dancing blew into my mind.

———————— • ————————

June. The time for the summer festival at Hemis Monastery renowned for its dancing monks. They commemorate the exorcism of age-old gods and the triumph of Buddhism over the Bön magicians. In the eighth century, the King of Tibet had trouble subduing the old beliefs, and he called in Padmasambhava, a Kashmiri sage and missionary, who, mastering the Shamans' tricks, used their magic to dispel demons in the name of the Buddha but being a wise, and wily man, for reasons of politics and doctrine, he gave space for the old gods in the Buddhist pantheon, and made the blood-drinking devils the guardians of the nether regions.

We rise early. The still cool valley is jammed with pilgrims and the buzz of voices. We cross the river and walk with the throng into the courtyard of the monastery. Crowds settle on the ground, and on top of the surrounding walls and the parapets. Others find places on the roof, and a handful of Europeans press their way into a two-storied arcade facing the monastery. The monks, packed onto the steps leading to the main temple, leave just enough room for the procession to come out. The drone increases with the hour, and I turn from one group to another, watching Indian women in dazzling saris, Ladakhis in dark velvet and heavy jewellery. A blind man accompanied by a boy playing a flute, hobbles along bent over a stick, his free hand twirling a prayer wheel. The child darts off to a group of tribal women in magnificent paraks. They keep to themselves; their men are busy elsewhere with friends and monks. In contrast to the women's traditional attire, youths from Leh strut the scene in jeans, while nobility, housed in the monastery, exit from dark doorways to take their stand on the balconies. It is pointless to ask when the dancing will begin; it will happen in its own good time.

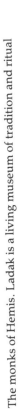

The monks of Hemis. Ladak is a living museum of tradition and ritual

A sudden shrill wail of cornets and the thud of drums hush the crowd. Out into the blazing sunlight comes Ladakh's cultural heritage in a medieval parade headed by the old Abbot escorted under a yellow silk canopy. Monks in brocades and rich head-dresses (strangely reminiscent of the Catholic Church) swing gilded bronze incense burners. Dancers appear in golden masks. Others in multicoloured robes prance with demon heads larger than their own. Shamans in aprons strung with human bones shake rattles. The hiss commands silence. The people watch, absorbed by the dancers' hypnotic movements in a slow round broken by short, ungainly jumps.

Normally, the monks spend days in retreat preparing themselves in meditation to invoke the spirits they will portray. This morning, I wonder how much of the ceremony is truly religious and how much has been staged for the few European visitors. I turn to a German next to me and ask what he thinks it is all about. 'The mystical connotation of the ceremonies we witness depicts the phantoms of the psyche slain in the arena of the heart before man can be released from reincarnation in this world of pain.' Really? I leave him to his erudite books and his pomposity.

On the second day, a yellow-robed monk in stag head-dress falls to the earth in a final spasm. I turn again to my German acquaintance. 'The death of the beast,' he says, 'represents the annihilation of selfishness. The ego is absorbed into the light of the Buddha.' On hearing his reply, an English speaking Ladakhi titters. 'it's far less complicated and much more practical.' he whispers. 'It's curtains for the demon inside the stag.'

On comes a giant figure, an incarnation of Padmasambhava under the name of Shawa, the Magician. His black mask, horns and fangs make him a veritable creature of a disturbed mind. He cuts to bits a human effigy made from dough . . . Everyone cheers. The mighty Buddha has triumphed. Padmasambhava has exorcised the devils with their own weapons.

Our sense of time is much more urgent than the Ladakhis. After the first hour, the majority of the foreigners were getting restless, bored and irritated by the repetitive movements, the slow pace of events that only twenty minutes earlier had mes-merised and enraptured them with their colour and exoticism. The gods and devils were just masked men in gorgeous dress who take their time in unfolding the plot of a heathen dance-pantomime. For them legend is bogged down in linear time instead of being perceived in the circle of an eternal chain of events woven with myth, a living force made vivid by roles that have a permanence – if not the mortals who play them. Do the Europeans think Padmasambhava is a Himalayan St George, the Dragon Slayer? The deities or the heroes of Ladakh do not destroy demons. One diverts the power of the other. The aim is to restore balance, not annihilate.

I watch the performers. They live in a flow of time that passes over immutable archetypes consecrated as inspirational roles for men to imitate, identify with and thus participate in the divine. I sympathise with the Ladakhis' attention to the drama's significance. I am thrilled aesthetically and captured the same way as by good theatre. Yet participation and identification elude me. I can't put my finger on the reason for this. The mystic convergence of self with images, static or animate, relies on a inexplicable and spontaneous alchemy of emotion that fuses your spirit with what you see.

This was more or less exactly what had happened when I saw the statue of Poseidon in the Athens Museum. Exquisitely balanced, javelin poised, he was a perfect representative of the divine shaped as man for as long as there is need of a body. I stood transfixed. Poseidon's face, his eyes absent from their sockets, could be a mask hiding a god's humanity. The masks of gods now before me belong to a different order of beings from whom I recoil unless I can accept them as personifications of my baser nature. In a culture where magic and myth are totally real, and its experience is valued more highly than any other, my identification remains sterile and intellectual. I cheat myself of the experience.

———————————— • ————————————

I closed my eyes and saw again those Shamans turn and spin in dances extended into slow motion.

'Nazir, what do you remember most clearly from our time at Hemis?'

'Our bath in the river when we had left the monastery. We sat on a rock watching the Ladakhis walk away in ant trails from the poplar grove in the ravine, out over wasteland and back to their villages. That was the scene I liked best. There were no foreigners. It was like scraping away modern paint from an old canvas and seeing the real design.' And, in that design, the pilgrims nurtured the certainty that in the repetition of existence, rested the mystery and the promise of progression for ALL beings, visible and invisible.

Hemis had its own mysteries. During the first decade of this century, Notovitch, a Russian traveller, maintained he had discovered manuscripts in Pali telling of contact between the early Nazarenes and the Ladakhis. The Hemis documents were proved a forgery. However, no one has disproved the incident of the miraculous Buddha presiding in the main temple. In the last Chinese attack on Ladakh, the enormous statue was found with an ear broken and dripping blood. This only stopped at the end of the Sino-Indian war in 1962. At about the same time, the Abbot of Phyang Monastery left his finger mark imprinted on a rock. The Chinese, he proclaimed, would not advance beyond that point. They did not.

We went on with our reminiscences. 'You know, last year I was back in Hemis. It's changed! There's a resthouse for busloads of tourists now. It's become an attraction just as we knew it would. I left the people I was with and went to look for our old camp. I found it, and stood there thinking of so many things.'

Both mountaineer and mechanic, Nazir was at heart a nomad. In his contact with Indians and Europeans, each trip furnished the rooms of his mind with memories, and under his brusqueness he hid a nostalgia for time spent with friends. I had often watched him stand apart in a monastery or on a mountain, and knew that he was reliving the past, recalling the conversations and the fun that he had enjoyed with his clients.

In silence we listened to the gusts of wind about us die in gasps. We opened the tent to see a valley clear of dust clouds and free from the wind's pestering. A goat bleated in the company of young voices calling in the thin air. 'Everything appears so normal doesn't it?' said Nazir, arms up and back arched in a long stretch. He rose and went out onto the grass. 'You wouldn't think there could be any nasty spirits lurking around here!'

'What's on your mind?'

'I once spent a night in a farmhouse in a place called Achrik, Two families live there with a hot spring and fields of millet. It's a magnificent setting in the mountains, as lovely and peaceful as this valley, only more remote. In the house, they had the usual nook in the wall for a private chapel. Only in this instance, it housed an evil god. His statue had been there for many generations, head always covered with a white cloth except for once a year when it was unveiled after two days of prayer. Every day the family carried a bowl of smoking pine needles through the house.' Nazir shivered.

'Did you believe in the magic?'

'Yes, because the place gave me the creeps. They told me not to sleep with my feet towards the idol. Heaven forbid! I knew that already. It's a sign of rudeness to gods and host, but you know me, I disregarded the custom for once, just to annoy the old boy, and had nightmares, horrible ones, the whole night long. Then my old host tried to scare me witless with the tall tale of a European who had sneaked into his house and removed the veil. He went bananas. Now, I will finish with another magical tale; a nice one. One of his boys played a double flute with six holes. It was really good listening to him trill away. It took forty-five minutes before a yak he had lost came down the mountain unshepherded with a few goats trailing behind.'

Enough of dark powers! We walked to the river and sat on the banks where the swirl passed over the rocks and curved its course into the distance; a land of Shamans and Buddhists, of Moslems, Christians and itinerant foreigners. At one time, Ladakh and the Zangskar were part of the Kushan Empire. At its height it stretched from Kashmir to the Punjab, from the frontiers of Bengal to Baluchistan, Afghanistan, and portions of Turkestan. Dominant at the time of Christ, the Kushans were thought to have been of Scythian stock from the steppes of Central Asia. When their greatest warrior emperor was converted to Buddhism, he settled in the north-west at the junction of four civilizations and among people familiar with Græco-Roman culture that had come with commerce. Cross pollination was inevitable. Mediterranean medicine left its mark and was itself influenced through contact with Buddhism.

To the east of the Kushans, lay the Han Empire. By the end of the second century, AD, Buddhism had reached China by way of trade with the Kushans. Along the silk routes threading the Middle Kingdom to the West, rose the Central Asian monasteries; Buddhist strongholds for pilgrims and scholars.

'Those camel caravans were extraordinary,' said Nazir, 'imagine travelling for months, sometimes years, moving along at just two and a half miles and hour. It gives me a backache just to think of it. How the monasteries must have been welcome sights!'

One of the historic stop-overs was at Tun-Huang, the last town on the western Chinese frontier. Its name means 'The Blazing Beacon', later changed to 'The Oasis in the Sand'. Twelve miles out from the oasis, in cliffs above the river, shrines cut into the rock sheltered objects and priests in periods of war and persecution. Tun-Huang grew prosperous. It received many intellectual impulses from East, West and South. Monks gathered manuscripts in the *lingua franca* of Sanskrit, and occupied themselves in translation. During the eleventh century AD, when the inhabitants anticipated an invasion from the southern tribes of Tibetan origin, the great library was walled up and only refound in 1907 by Sir Aurel Stein, the British scholar-explorer. The library contained the first block-printed book dated approximately to 868 AD. It proved to be the most ancient document of purely Tibetan origin, written in the seventh century. Its contents deal with Tibet's pre-Buddhic culture, and described Bön rituals, exorcism, divination of disease and veterinary care for horses. No reference is made to any herbal, mineral or vegetable substances for drugs. From this, experts deduced that there was only the most rudimentary medical knowledge before Vedic scripts were brought to Tibet by the Buddhist missionaries.

Marco Polo, a devout Catholic, visited the caves as an envoy of Kublai Khan, the grandson of Ghengis. Despite his long years in the East, he had little sympathy for Buddhism. For him, Buddhists were devil worshippers. Thus he upheld the Khan's hidden predilection for Christianity even though he noted that the old emperor, already in his eighties, feared the Shamans' necromancy and hoped for the arrival of Catholic priests armed with a power demontratively greater than their rivals. Marco Polo gives accounts of the magicians' control over weather and the levitation of goblets automatically filled with wine. If he was impressed by their magic, he still described the Shamans as filthy and indecent, some of whom consumed the cremated flesh of criminals in order to foster their supernatural power. Furthermore, he observed that exorcism for illness was common practice in Cathay, a physician was rare, and 'sported with the blindness of deluded and wretched people'.

Night fell, the quiet disrupted by the howls of a few dogs. We returned to camp for dinner. Before sleep, my spirit flew out to the domains of Shamans and great caravans where I heard the bells on camels' feet, and bathed in Oriental mysteries, I went into dreams.

NOTE

[1] Menstrual blood contains oestrogen, arsenic, lecithine and cholesterol.

SEVEN

—————————•—————————

We visit a psychic healer trained by the Lamas

A VISIT TO THE LHA-MO

The air was exceptionally clear, and snow had fallen on the peaks. 'Look!' I called, pointing towards the mountain. I was caught up by the contagious laughter coming from a gang of children, several with fat, Buddha-babies bouncing on their backs as they yelped and jumped down the slopes from Karsha. The youngsters clamoured for pictures. Laughter everywhere. Fun and games. Songs sung anew. I had forgotten the delights of such simple things.

'I am I and you are you,' say the texts, 'and the universe is within us. I participate in your feelings, you in mine.'

I was less willing to apply these easy, happy thoughts of our autumn days to the snow-bound bitterness of winter. In that season of discomfort, the Amchi, his own living conditions hardly better than his patients, would make his rounds to the sick and the healthy huddled in houses reeking of smoke, acrid and thick from burning dung with little heat. It damaged the lungs and eyes.

Sonam had never boasted of any spectacular cure. He had, in the progress of his visits, acquainted us with his medicine and the philosophy that Ignorance and spiritual blindness pierced by desire, drew humans into the stress that rebounded on their constitution. In Ladakh, sheer physical survival required a strong desire to stay with the flesh.

Just before seven o'clock on that fine morning, Sonam strode into camp. The burgundy robe hit by the sun and that gliding, measured walk could belong to no other than him.

'The Amchi cometh!' We went to escort our man of medicine into the mess tent. He was in fine form and full of humour in his talk with Nazir. He accepted a handful of dried apricots, then, with a wave of his hand, commanded our departure.

'Cumweego!' he said. A surprise, he repeated, awaited us in a village not far away. We were off to see a 'Lha-mo'. Sonam explained the word. 'Lha' referred to someone who was 'a representative of the gods', a person with 'the breath of divinity'. Lha-mo was the feminine form.

'So! we're off to see a Shaman,' I exclaimed.

'You might call her that,' Nazir replied, 'but Sonam tells me she is rather special and was trained by the chief Lama attached to the Royal Household.'

Her mother, also a psychic, had reincarnated seven times into the same family. When she died, her five year-old daughter was noted to have the same calling, and the child's abnormal behaviour, heightened in adolescence, confirmed her disposition. The priests decided to take over her education and occult training.

Shamans have intuitive, mercurial personalities. Some are epileptics or carry the defects of six fingers or more teeth than normal. Marked for their vocation, they await the onslaught of spirit voices and hallucination that western doctors dismiss as the products of fear reinforced by traditions. Be this as it may, they suffer physical and psychic agonies. Initiations plunge them into the terror of having to subdue the elemental beings of their mythology. The 'lha' of a Shaman can enter beasts for combat with the demons inhabiting other animals, and the winner's power is assured when he or she has overcome the opponent's will. As an ultimate test, they go into a coma and experience excruciating forms of death from which they return qualified to divine and heal. Psychics, according to Buddhism, are vessels for powers which, if not released, can cause schizophrenia and even suicide. Mediums in an altered state of consciousness demolish the distinction between the inner and outer realities. They 'ride the Pulse of Life' and become what they see. Alternatively, powers can from time to time take over the Shaman. In the flux of change nothing stays permanent in shape or character. Beasts are inhabited by humans and humans by gods or demons. The initiate achieves his ends through ritual, ecstasy, concentration and visualisation.

In an hour we came to the village. On reaching a freshly whitewashed house, a softly spoken man in his fifties welcomed us at the door. He was the Lha-mo's husband and father of her five children. With the usual Ladakhi consideration for travellers, he showed us up the stairs into a room where we could wash our hands and faces.

A woman of undefinable age darted in, spoke with Sonam, flashed a brilliant smile in our direction, and went off, swift as a bird. She left the impression of a most vital and organised person about her daily chores, and like so many Ladakhis, radiated good humour that bubbles up from their inner resources. She was the Lha-mo, and had arranged to see us in about half an hour after completing her morning prayers. The house, the neatest and newest I had seen, had only been built within the last year.

'She's made a lot of money from Europeans and Indians; enough for new rooms and the beautiful wooden windows,' said Nazir. No wonder she exuded such self-confidence. Even after our short encounter, I was struck by her incisive air and normality; her eyes had none of that wild look of the village Shamans. She was, added Sonam, quite undisturbed by spirits unless in a deliberate trance. The locals considered her as an expeller of demons rather than an Amchi. Her first duty was to restore the stolen life force, and she acted in the fashion of their legendary heroes; an intermediary between the visible and the unseen.

Shamanism mixed with Buddhism is taken for granted, and like the medieval alchemist, Paracelsus, Ladakhis accepted illness as a kind of purgatory. In every sickness there rested a crisis of conscience leading to purification. The Lha-mo intervened at a requested moment to take responsibility for a cure, helped when the patient participated with faith, itself a type of initiation.

'Do people have to have unquestioned faith in the Lha-mo's for her cures to work?' I asked.

The Amchi rubbed his chin in a familiar gesture. 'She heals cows and goats that have swallowed stones or pieces of tin, and if the owner is not sure of her powers, I have seen her make the object rise half way out of the flesh before letting it sink back again. I leave you to make up your own mind.'

'Can she tell the future?'

'If you want to know, why not ask her yourself,' chuckled Sonam. Our discussion was interrupted by the Lha-mo's husband. He came in with a tray of tea and biscuits. We sat on the floor sipping, munching and smelling the incense from the chapel in the room next door.

'My wife is a very devout person,' said our host, 'she prays every day before working with up to twenty patients. Healing makes her very tired. She sleeps in the afternoons.' He smiled shyly and left the room.

'The Lamas usually restrain trained women psychics from public healing until they are forty and have preferably raised a family,' said Sonam. 'Last year, a Japanese doctor came here. The Lha-mo sucked out his kidney stones through his solar plexus. He went off a most happy man, taking his relics with him. We judge the power of each Lha by the number of spirits that communicate through them, and our Lha-mo is one of the best. Four divinities speak from her mouth . . . each with a different voice'.

Asian Shamans say their 'lha' is taken by spirits and guided to other realms, or that it rides the back of the animal whose skin is stretched across their drums. In Ladakh, mediums insist to the contrary. The spirits descend. The 'lha' does not fly away with a guide. On our host's return, we went down to the kitchen where his wife prepared herself for consultation.

The atmosphere was pregnant with expectancy. Red turbaned Sikhs from Padum crushed against dust covered farmers and peasants stinking of goat. Indian women in saris stood beside young monks whispering prayers and fingering beads. In the gloomy room, a ray of light from a single window struck the Lha-mo's blue and silver brocade cape and the sapphire blue Buddha of medicine painted on the central panel of her head-dress with five coloured ribbons. If one fell, it foretold her death. She intermittently rattled a small, double-headed drum in one hand. The other held a bell rung in high chimes against the steady chant as she recited in front of the altar alongside the stove.

In the web of micro–macro relationships, her body was a receptacle for the supernatural. With her head-dress, her drum and the ritual gestures she made to the cardinal points, colour, sound and direction invoked a spirit's association with the human realm. A child wailed uncontrollably in distress muffled against its mother's belly. She jiggled it up and down on her lap. No one paid any attention. Hers was the only movement in the crowd. All the others, standing or kneeling, were lost in concentration, faces turned to the Lha-mo, their eyes wide and glazed, or closed, prepared for what still escaped me . . . mystical participation.

Into that taut anticipation came a hen. It cautiously pecked its way across the dirt floor to stalk around my feet. An ordinary occurrence, I thought, in a farmhouse kitchen. But the bird was far from ordinary. A blue streak of paint ran down its back. I nudged Nazir.

'Don't worry about that now,' he murmured, 'Shamans have their familiar spirits, just like a witch's cat. Leave our lady's feathered friend alone and pretend you haven't noticed it.' His advice made me think of my nurse, who, with the dignity of a duchess used to say 'Stop looking at that silly man or he won't go away'. The hen, looked at or not, clucked away in its territorial imperative.

The Lha-mo abruptly pivoted round from the altar, picked up a thin, wooden baton, and tapping the first patient on the shoulder, an Indian woman, uttered a spate of words in a high, testy voice. Rapidly delivered, they were the words of someone compelled to say a great deal in a short time. The transformation was startling. One moment she had chanted prayers in her normal pitch, and the next she spoke in an absolutely altered tonality. Nonetheless, her change in voice and manner was the same as any medium taken over in trance by another personality. Nazir stood next to me in the semi-darkness. 'She's telling the woman her fortune. It sounds a bit vague to me. Her Urdu is not so hot, but all the nods must mean the lady agrees.' The stream of words ceased as quickly as it had begun. The Lha-mo pointed her stick within half an inch of the woman's jugular vein, and sucking the other end for a few seconds, spat out a gob of black mucus into a silver bowl. The stick, used to withdraw 'poisons' from above the chest, symbolised the Shaman's Tree of Life joining the lower to the higher worlds; but a medium can employ any sacred object as a conductor for a divinity's power.

She rinsed her mouth with saffron water, and swung round again, this time to a Ladakhi. He raised his shirt, and after a short conversation, the Lha-mo bent to place her lips on his solar plexus. Moments later, she removed from her mouth a pea-sized black blob. Pulled apart with her fingernails, it released an inordinate amount of grey slime. It was, she explained a grain of cursed rice. Now that she had removed the cause of his stomach pain, she said he had better give prayers of thanks and ask the Buddha to protect him from his enemies.

Before I had time to refuse, Nazir whispered, 'Your turn! Kneel down, shut up and I will tell her you suffer from watery eyes.' Torn between curiosity and scepticism, I let him push me onto my knees.

Her lips, light as a dragonfly, touched my solar plexus. The feeling was strange. The pressure, quite negligible, gave me the sensation that my flesh itself was fluttering more than responding to exterior suction. I felt as if its density changed with atoms momentarily re-arranged, and firm matter stretched and rendered

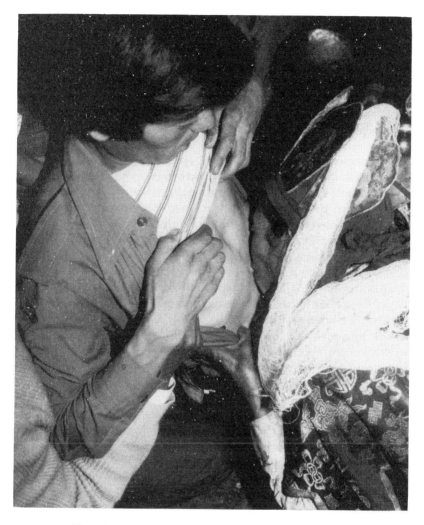

The Lhamo extracts poison from a client's diaphragm

porous became a membrane through which the Lha-mo withdrew the black substance she spewed into the bowl beside her. The whole procedure had taken but half a minute. Eyes lowered, she pronounced in a high voice that I suffered from 'bad blood', and no more could be done in this first session. She rinsed out her mouth and covered her lips with ash before attending to the next person.

'Please come with me,' I sighed to Nazir, 'I want to get out of here and examine my stomach.' Outside, Nazir and I examined the faintly pink mark left on the skin where the Lha-mo had put her mouth. Around it lay a light aureole of ash. The delicate pressure she had applied, I was convinced could not have withdrawn any liquid nor left the mark on my skin. I had none of the mucous to analyse. Perhaps she had regurgitated it, and kept a supply of ash in her mouth. The ash came from burnt animal bones, and was a disinfectant. We had seen her smear it over her lips, and with a sleight of hand she might have slipped other substances into her mouth at the same time. First rate conjurers are known to duplicate psychic phenomena, but what of the Japanese doctor's kidney stones carried home for discussion on the method of their removal and proof that they were his and not a conjurer's replacement? Moreover, they could have disintegrated as had been reported from Brazil and the Philippines where psychic healers materialise matter for a limited duration. I was reluctant to condemn the Lha-mo as a fraud, and disregarding the unchanged state of my eyes, I felt exceptionally well and recharged with vigour. My shirt tucked back into place, I returned to the kitchen.

Now at the end of her seance, the Lha-mo was giving homage to the five senses in a classic ritual. Her chants, delivered in her normal voice, reminded the gathering of their faculty for hearing. The grain thrown about drew attention to taste, the incense and altar decorated with flowers recalled the sense of smell and sight. Her touch had already eased their minds and who knows what psychosomatic disturbances had been withdrawn. I had witnessed a magico-medical performance offering psychotherapy in a social event where, while she worked on one patient, the others became conditioned for their own cures.

I called softly to Sonam when he appeared from upstairs. He waited by the door and we passed out into the courtyard to join Nazir dozing in the sunshine. I was disappointed. My eyes had not improved. 'Is it because my heart wasn't in it?' I asked Sonam.

'Heart! That is the important word,' he said, 'but I mean your physical organ. Your eyes, you told me, have troubled you for years, every time you are in dusty places. The poison in your blood has flowed through your heart for far too long. The Lha-mo could not cure you straight off; your condition is better treated by an Amchi. The cure is long.' Sonam believed in her cures in so far as she manipulated matter in a way he could not duplicate. For all his expertise, he in turn was astute enough to recognise the value of surgery in Leh for cases beyond his ability.

The medical rounds in Ladakh went from Shaman to Priest to Amchi and finally, to the government clinics. Whatever the method of healing, if one was not successful, there were alternatives. The range of options, rational and irrational, fitted in with the Buddhist creed which kept a place for 'the all-identifying magic mind' that ignores a fractured psyche. The lamas were also canny enough to take in gifted mediums and never alienated the people from their grass roots traditions.

Magic, a vague term not rigorously defined, thank goodness, is ambiguous, unusual, marginal and transitional. Magic, a state of being and becoming directed by its own laws, is as if space, time and events are muddled together and put into a crucible called 'The Supernatural', where, reduced to chaos, they are reassembled to emerge apparently as before; yet altered. Now was the moment to question Sonam about the hen.

'That hen with the blue stripe along its back; was it the Lha-mo's familiar spirit?' asked Nazir, his face quite serious. The Amchi lowered his eyes. His answer was indirect.

'In the Shaman's fourth heaven,' he said, 'among other gods and benevolent deities, lives the "Lady of the White Hen", a protectress for women children and childbirth. Auxiliary spirits, never harmful when from these spheres, can inhabit a domestic animal, bird, or close friend who might also be a sexual partner.'

Priestess-healer-seer, the Lha-mo's functions flowed one into the other, and from her monastic training, she was regarded as one cut above the other Shamans, benign or evil, with their filtres for seducing maidens, and copper mirrors to divine the future. She was revered to a same extent as the Lama/Exorcists, mediums called upon to banish earth demons and to bless the soil in spring and before harvests.

Ladakh is a living museum. Priests, resplendent in silks, swords lifted above their heads, dance in trance along the parapets of a monastery, and with the sixth sense of a somnambulist, miss tumbling to their deaths. I had watched one Lama, a renowned medium, mounted on a white stallion, ride out from the monastery to bless the fields. The procession, a surging sea of maroon and black, passed over the land and on to a chorten where he had leapt, robes flapping in the white heat like a phoenix in defence of its sacred nest.

One winter, a friend on a photographic assignment in Ladakh covered a series of religious festivals. In one monastery, he and other photographers were warned against taking pictures of masked priests during a certain stage of the dancing. None took the threat seriously. My friend sensibly remained apart and shot his pictures under cover leaving his colleagues to fire away blatantly until a Lama, possessed behind his horrific mask, charged straight at them, sword raised. They ran. Shortly afterwards, all except my friend, were brought low by strange illnesses and bad luck. One died. Months later, the incident well out of mind, my friend, was walking with his slides stacked in a carousel firmly closed in a box under his arm. He slipped. The box rose into the air, opened and disgorged its contents into the gutter filled with water. It was, he described, as if in that moment, he floated in time, watching the scene in slow motion, powerless to move.

Shaman, Priest and Amchi, each had their place in healing. But since no standardisation regulates their practice, results range from incompetence to the learned therapies of traditional doctors. Today, medical choice for the population is widened with clinics and western drugs. East turns West, West looks to the Orient, and along old routes come new caravans of thought from Europe interested in quantifying ancient prescriptions and esoteric cures.

A HOLISTIC EXPERIENCE

We left the Lha-mo's house and trod the narrow track back to camp. The men soon outpaced me, and immured in my thoughts, when I looked up, Nazir and the Amchi were already far ahead on the pastures. From the heights every component of the land-scape had its ordained place. Nature spread itself in front of me, and from behind the beauty, and beyond words or reason, came an immense replenishment that sustained my existence. I stood seized by the wonder I had sought on leaving Paris for the Hima-layas.

One can read, talk, listen, but only when thoughts are felt do they pass from the reality of others into one's own personal universe. Now, without prior warning, emotion had condensed my shifting mood into a magic moment of wholeness in which, despite Buddhist theory on the illusion of the self, I was extended into an unimaginable eternity. The happening gave me a first hand experience, however meagre, of Sonam's explanation of matter when he had said: 'Things are objects of knowledge ... they are not independent of an enquirer.'

On looking out across the landscape, the rock underfoot had

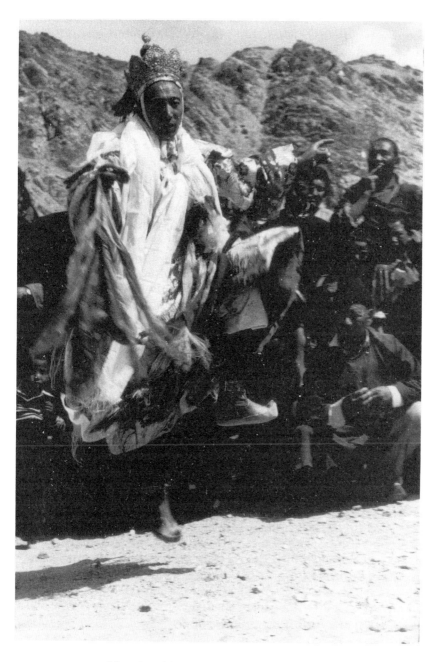

A leaping abbot dances at a harvest festival

become as intangible as thought itself. It indicated no static point. Time was no longer something that marked the measure of my steps through space. My relationship with my senses had altered, and in the transformation they had fused into one extrasensory organ that obliterated normal differentiation between what my eyes saw, my ears heard, my skin felt, or my mind made real. My skin, that sevenfold casing, had expanded, and with it, my shape embraced all I beheld. Inadvertently, I had fallen into a perception common to Shamans; a faculty as ancient as man himself, but once experienced, never to be called 'primitive'. I had come full circle back to that moment when, aged ten, and spellbound by the sun's eclipse, my apprehension of some awesome power had projected me into a new relationship with the desert. At the time it was more than my intellect could cope with, but I knew that henceforth the world would not always be as it appeared, for behind the profane lay the sacred.

I still could not fathom what had unleashed these feelings. The shift from everyday perception into another awareness was as spontaneous as had been my confrontation with Poseidon. The only added factor was my contact with the Lha-mo. Had she, in 'cleansing my blood' actually cleared the subtle channels of my mind? In this case, cause was secondary to effect.

SONAM DEALS WITH TWO INFECTIONS

I reached camp to find Sonam examining the tiny capillaries behind the ear of a sick baby held in its mother's arms. The infant's wrists were too small for pulse reading. 'The Amchi say it's got mumps, poor thing,' Nazir informed me, puffing out his cheeks. The baby's face, as yet unswollen, was wet with sweat.

'The fever is an infectious one, and fanned by the Wind Nopa it is spreading,' said Sonam, 'I will make bone soup with diluted camphor, bamboo manu, white sandalwood and rock sugar. I need to be vigilant and watch the reaction before I can adjust the compound. No formula is increased or decreased too quickly. The soup I use as a test. It draws out the symptoms, especially for the Wind. Camphor is the king of fever medicines, a savage monarch who needs guidance from good counsellors. His chief minister is Sandalwood. I can add up to twenty-five other ingredients to the king/ minister compound which tames the basic mixture, otherwise Camphor's cold nature blows the fever into a fire.'

Sonam described the treatment of chronic, ripe, unripe, hidden, turbid and many other qualities of fevers in pungent analogies such as 'wet wood exuding smoke before the flame,' or 'when the mountain meets the plain – the stage when a subsided fever leaves the underlying disease to manifest itself. The doctor is the archer. He chooses his arrow, the hot or cold potency of the medicine, diet and therapy, and targets it on one or a combination of imbalanced Nopas. Sonam handed the mother his preparations, and with a nod she was away, no payment offered.

Sonam accepted our invitation for a late lunch. As we were about to sit, Gulam, our cook, head down and wiping his hands on the edge of his stained shirt, walked halfway towards us, caught Nazir's eyes, and called him with a jerk of his head. After talking behind the tent, they returned to Sonam. Gulam, stubborn as a goat and without a tongue to boot, pulled up his shirt to let a large boil on his back speak for itself.

'He's terrified the Amchi will cut him,' said Nazir with little sympathy.

'No! I am not afraid. Praise be to Allah!' cried Gulam in English, having refound his vocal cords. 'You are wrong Nazir.'

'Then what's the matter man? For God's sake speak to the Amchi, he understands Urdu.'

Sonam probed around the boil. Gulam flinched saying, again in English, 'This funny man is going to tell me I can't eat curry and red peppers. He will order me to swallow bowls of that foul grey porridge. I can't eat their food. It makes me sick.'

'Well, tell him so, you idiot. I'm not translating for you,' said Nazir, laughing. But our zealous cook mislaid his tongue once more. Sonam prescribed a medicine and paste he would prepare that evening and send with Thelmy the next morning. The boil should clear up in four days; no lancing necessary. Meantime, Gulam had better refrain from his usual food and endless cups of strong tea laced with the condensed milk further sweetened with white sugar, so dear to his taste. Nazir reached into his pocket. The Amchi raised his hand in protestation, and Gulam slunk back to his pots.

The texts state a doctor's right to prosperity gained from good motives. Sonam had no desire to secure wealth. The Lha-mo earned far more than he did. His riches came from meritorious acts. He lived by the laws of Dharma, and each day, withdrew to meditate[1] on his actions. But what was the true self of Sonam Gyelsen of Karsha? His inner identity came from elements whose association gave birth to his temporary being. Instant by instant they altered, but his awareness gave the impression of an ego since the body permitted sensation, perception and mental activity and thus self-consciousness. Sonam, although an individual brought into a series of lives on earth, had no eternal identity. He was part of the universal equation that emanated from a mysterious First Cause.

After a second cup of coffee that Sonam said he should not drink but could not resist, he proposed a visit to his master in the monastery, or if the Abbot preferred, a meeting in Sonam's house. He rose, shook hands and strode from the camp.

'He's become our alter ego. I always feel deprived when he leaves.' I said, watching his figure diminish in the distance. Sonam came and went on the wind.

NOTES

[1] The root of the word meditate is 'med'. It comes from the Latin word to make, look after or heal. In the same way, 'meditation' was once intimately connected with 'medicine'. The word 'physician' is rooted in the ancient word 'bheu' meaning nature itself, then the Greek 'phusis'. Thus meditation, medicine, nature and physician retain their old associations.

EIGHT

We meet the Amchi's Lama-master—He discusses death, healing, esoteric practices and answers questions on Tibet

A PREMONITION OF DEATH

It was a morning when the sun seemed to bathe the valley in a golden elixir. Yet, eating breakfast on the grass, I had a presentiment of death that brought goosepimples to my arms. Alice, my friend with terminal cancer, I felt sure had died. I said so to Nazir.

'What makes you think such a thing?'

'I don't know.' Nothing backed up my hunch except the sorrow passing through me. For months, bedridden Alice had injected morphine into her bloated stomach. Parties were frequent. We came with food and wine and went in and out of her bedroom until she fell asleep. Her will to live, her wish to be of use to others, never waned. Life she had faced. Death had been ignored.

Alice committed outrageous, self-defeating acts that were as wilful as her courage. As a confirmed atheist, Sonam's belief in countless existences would have slid from her like quicksilver from a steely mask of feigned interest. I wondered what fears were to be her ultimate companions. Perhaps in her denial of an afterlife, she had hoped to short-circuit Christian tenets of redemption, the last judgement or the intervention of divine grace to ease retribution. I doubted if she would have even wanted the Buddhist choice of a new chance on earth denied to Christians, but at the hard core of the Buddha's compassion lay the teaching that we, and we alone are responsible for our evolution. He exhorted his disciples to be their own light and their own refuge.

'It's a shame Alice is not with us.' I said half to myself.

'Are you saying that the Amchi could have helped her?'

'Partly. Tibetans have a positive attitude towards death, and some Lamas in the West are interpreting their Book of the Dead in ways most helpful to the terminally ill and those near them.' The texts describe the sensations accompanying death and the release of the unconsciousness into an unfamiliar state. The descriptions have a remarkable similarity to near death experiences recorded in the West. Different cultures have different images, but, by and large, we all appear to travel through darkness towards light in which some figure awaits our arrival. Some report finding themselves on a railway station without timetable or luggage, and filled with angst they know no more than they must catch a train to an unknown destination.

Our melancholic mood left us when our gang of children came jogging into camp, and all smiles, they planted themselves strategically outside the mess tent for Gulam and Mohamet to hand out chapattis and a large, communal mug of coffee. They all learn the rudiments of reading and writing from Sonam's eldest son, the school master. Ceremonies of life and death were part of their upbringing. The mysteries of dying, however, and the states between incarnations belong to the scriptures taught in monastic communities. Mystic secrets were not for the laity. Esoteric knowledge was for the priests who, in theory, were expected to have a moral distinction equivalent to their learning.

'Nazir!' I called, 'I promised Alice I'd open a bottle of champagne on her death. Let's do the next best thing and fill our mugs with tea, call the kids and have a good sing song.'

We assembled the gang, and soon they were belting out the finest rendition of their favourite ditties.

'To Alice!' we shouted.

'May she fly away from sorrow speeded along on the breath of song', called Nazir, raising his mug to the sky.

Unexpectedly, the Amchi's voice joined ours. He stood beaming, hand on his beads, and when told the reason for the concert, nodded his approval. All thoughts, he said, had power. I gave him a resume of Alice's cancer. First found in her breast, it had followed the Tibetan theory that disease enters by way of the skin into the flesh, travels in the blood and drops into the internal organs moving on to consume the bones.

'If you are right in feeling your friend has left this realm, her death, I hope you understand, has importance and meaning. Nothing in life is meaningless. All is change, so please, no sadness, that will not help her departed 'lha'. Just think of her with deep, peaceful love', counselled Sonam, his eyes wide and relaxed in sympathy. 'Be happy! My master, the Rinpoche, is coming to my house this evening.

One of the main differences between the Buddhist and Christian doctrine is their approach to emotion. The Christian tries to spiritualise emotion. But the rapture of Christian love is too intense for the Buddhists. They learn to control emotion in search of wisdom and the equilibrium of detachment. I once saw this beautifully put into practice in America.

A Lama assembled round him about a dozen people. He picked on one woman in particular, and urged her to talk about her deepest problems. Since she hoped to gain the attention and sympathy of all those in the room, she began to pour out her troubles, no details spared. Five minutes went by. The Lama turned to another, 'Please, continue, I'm listening', he said to the woman, but persuaded the second person to talk at the same time. Soon, in a chorus conducted by the Lama, everyone was unloading their sorrows simultaneously, until suddenly aware of the situation, a young man burst out laughing. The Lama, having made his point, led the group into a crescendo of mirth that took them out of their utter self-absorption.

'Here, honoured Amchi!' called Nazir from the mess tent. He came out with a cup of coffee. 'This may pollute your blood but I know you will like it. By the way, Gulam's boil is doing nicely. The paste has worked wonders, but don't believe him if he says he's given up curries. He hasn't, they're hot to the point of eruption and I smell them on his breath.' The two of them went off to find our obstinate cook.

'How was he?' I asked.

'Gulam had paralysis of the tongue', answered Nazir. 'He's impossibly stubborn and refused to answer any of Sonam's questions directly. He simply gazed skywards muttering to Allah until I kicked him in the shins and made him talk. He admitted he had drunk the mixture which, he said, was distilled from an unmentionable ancestry of demonic substances.'

'We always tell our patients', added Sonam, 'that the nastier the taste, the better the results.' With a smile and a reminder of our meeting at sundown, he walked off. The sight of his erect figure moving across the landscape called to mind the unique way in which the Tibetans view their land.

Nearly twelve centuries ago, a manuscript discovered in the caves of Tun Huang, recounts the myth of Tibet's first king, and his descent from the sky:

> He came as Lord of the six regions of Tibet, and when he first arrived on earth, he came as the master of all that is found under the limits of the sky. From the centre of heaven to the midst of earth, at the heart of the continent girdled by snows, head of all waters, pure ground and high mountains. Excellent land . . . .

Space. Place. Centre. Each concept is defined and marked out. Each ecological zone has its connotations and is related in a strict hierarchy which, in its vertical scale, reflects the importance of height. Height, a value in itself, denotes the purest and the most esteemed state and the situation nearest the domain of the great gods residing in their heavenly realm above the mountains. Topped by eternal snow, the peaks are the home of mythical creatures; the white-breasted eagle and the wonderous white lioness with her turquoise mane. Below come the eyrie of other eagles, snow partridges and the ibex, followed by a zone of rocks embedded in clay running into Alpine pastures for antelope and wild, free animals. Between the opposition of mountains and valleys, lie high plateau roamed by wild yak and horses.

Each strata has its own particular species. Man, in the scheme of this landscape, gains merit according to his habitat. The pure hermit clings to the heights. The pilgrim, if he can, takes the most elevated path along the snow line to holy places. Likewise, in family and social hierarchy, the height of a seat denotes its importance, also marked by its position within the gathering centred around the main pillar of the room. To be centred both within oneself and the environment is the ideal situation. The mythical lioness should not leave her heights, nor the eagle his rocks, the fish its lake, nor man his chosen surroundings. He should stay in the place of his work or contemplation. The gods and divinities have their own centres, such as mountains, (which can become divinities themselves), from where they protect an area commensurate with their powers. Sky, mountains, earth and water spirits each have an alloted abode, the seat of their power from where they are invoked, honoured and propitiated. In this descending scale, Tibetans juxtapose the merits of the height to the baseness of low ground; the heart of things to the periphery. Everything is related to mankind composed of the same Elements that form the stratified landscape.

MEETING THE ABBOT

For the rest of that day, we idled in the sun, read and paddled in the river. We enjoyed the luxury of time that was ours to spend as we wished. When the sun fell behind the mountains, we walked to the Amchi's house carrying dried fruit and nuts, tea and sugar as gifts for the Rinpoche. We had no white gauze scarves, the traditional offerings for such an occasion. Sonam's room was lit with one lamp, and there, ensconced on a cushion on the bed, sat Rinpoche Tensing the Tulku.

Thelmy squatted on the floor. He jumped up and pulled from his robe two white scarves, and in turn we approached the master to lay them at his feet. He smiled politely. His gentle, modulated voice, his slow gestures, the composure of his presence and his lovely face were the epitome of what an elderly Tulku should be.

The scene, too perfect for my comfort, stripped me of all small talk, and left my mind a blank, I sat there ill at ease waiting for Sonam to start the conversation. No one said anything. Silence. The Amchi's sister came in with tea. Cups steamed in the silence. Sonam looked my way and nodded. I took a deep breath and hoped the action alone would pop a question into my head. Nothing happened. I shivered. Of course! 'Tun-mo', a method of raising the body's temperature by meditation and breath control. In a voice appropriately lowered to tune in with the Abbot's calm, I asked if this practice of drying-out wet sheets in sub-zero weather by wrapping them around a monk was taught in his monastery. I mentioned the American doctors in Daramsala who had measured a 15 degree Farenheit jump in the temperature of the body's extremities within 40 minutes from the start of meditation. Three monks had submitted to scientific analysis of a practice developed over six years of daily application in isolated, unheated, stone huts at the foot of the Himalayas.

The Lama-Amchi remained still, his expression remote until his shoulders shook and he brought his hand to his face. He sat vibrating with suppressed amusement, and addressing Sonam in a stifled voice, told him what he thought was so funny. Sonam's laugh, light and short, preceded the explanation. Westerners were inclined to be over impressed by extreme cases of mind dominating matter. It should not be given undue importance. Body heat was essential and needed for comfort in the winters and also for digestion, but, if you had no Tantric training, there was always the cat. Place it on your tummy, it was good for you and good for the cat, even if it ate your food before you did.

Tulku Tensing regained his composure and crossed his legs in the lotus position with the soles of his feet turned upwards. Elbows pressing into his insteps, he massaged the pressure points in the flesh between his thumbs and forefingers. Combined with breathing, this was a simple way of increasing the body's heat. Not to the extent of drying wet clothes, but enough for normal, practical purposes.

'Yes', he concluded, 'Tun-mo was still taught to purify the mind, but not as an exaggerated display of super-normal prowess.' We smiled, and passed round more tea. The Rinpoche handled his cup with the utmost delicacy. 'This evening, we have no need for Tun-mo or the cat', he said.

A DISCUSSION ABOUT DEATH

Without any prompting, Sonam opened the conversation on the nature of death. He told the Rinpoche that my friend had probably died, and asked him if he would give prayers for her journey into the Bardo. Tulku Tensing straightened his back. As the body dies, he said, the mind, no longer limited by the senses, becomes extremely clear, penetrating and clairvoyant. If the individual has been prepared for this event, it is a time when the greatest of all changes can occur; a moment of spiritual awakening providing the consciousness has relinquished worldly attachments.

Should doubt and fear arise, it can be used to advantage in an admission that habitual ways of thought and emotion need not be finite. Just after death, there may be a lightning vision of the supreme actuality and the opportunity for liberation. Karma, unluckily, usually draws us back into incarnation from the regions of the Bardo where condensation of thought forms crystallise into the matter of an earthly existence. There are, he explained, ways of meditation and techniques of visualisation most helpful for the dying.

'Visualise the sky before you with a Buddha, your Christ, a saint or your spiritual master in the full glory of a heavenly body. Give your consciousness the shape of a ball of light the size of an egg. Say the word "OM" quietly, and imagine the ball of light shooting out like a star from your heart to become one with the image. Consider your mind as one with your chosen, radiant image. Imagine this often for yourself or for the dying person, each time, three times over. When the mind is one with the image, remain still. This is the state of consciousness you should keep at the moment of death, just as the last breath leaves the body, it is the moment when Air dissolves into Space and with it come white, red and obscure visions. The white vision is like autumn moonlight caused by the vital force as it passes up the cool left hand channel of the mystic body to open the crown chakra. The second, copper-red vision arises as the life force ascends the hot, right channel to meet the central channel where they meet in the heart chakra.'

Death, he instructed us, is the reverse of life coming from the conjunction of the Elements. Dying is a process of separation. At a certain stage, it produces a vision of emptiness as the lower aspects of the mind fall asleep letting more refined perceptions awake. Confusion can be mastered, but due to karmic law, every past thought and action has its impact. Unless we have become proficient in spiritual practice, we are apt to decline into delusion. However, hopefully at death, muddled thoughts and emotions evaporate, and in the rupture from all familiar things, the dying can perceive a higher meaning to life.

'In the West', continued the Tulku, 'you do not recognise death's significance. You struggle on in ignorance and fear. One of our greatest sages and poets, Milarepa, said "My religion is not to be ashamed of myself when I die". When your consciousness has left the body, you are in a mental body of the Golden Age, complete with all your senses and none of the defects you might have had on earth. It is your vehicle in the Bardo for forty-nine days before your next existence. Movement anywhere is without obstruction, and travel happens by just thinking where you wish to go. Your awareness is nine times clearer, but, for the first four and a half days, before memories of the previous life fade, you can still see your loved ones on earth. Their weeping is like a thunderstorm, and any fights over inheritance upset you greatly. I know of one case where the departed one put a curse on his family. This is why we teach the bereaved to concentrate on positive things and remember that one good thought can change the existence of the wandering "lha" in the Bardo, especially during the first twenty-one days, because later it is drawn to its next state. It is never too late to pray for the departed or dedicate good deeds in his or her memory. Give me the name of your friend and I will offer guidance. Please, never try to contact those in the Bardo. It only hinders them.'

Suicide is an act of terrible ignorance – as if the Buddha principle within had been murdered. Family and friends should never judge the victim, but pray for his or her peace of mind and contact a master since that person may have died in great anger, sadness and delusion. The consciousness is then trapped with the body and becomes a ghost in the earth realm. On the seventh day after the suicide, prayers should be given at the same time as the death, and if possible in the same place.

Training in this life prepares one to combat the attractions of rebirth, or to choose rather than being irresistibly pulled into one of the six realms in the wheel of existence. Each realm is announced by colour. Visions appear. White for the gods in their domain of splendid temples in groves and palaces made of jewels. Red for the jealous deities and their revolving wheel of fire. Green for the animal state with scenes of caves and holes in the ground. Yellow for the hungry ghosts clinging to tree stumps and other dark shapes in caverns. The lowest realm has a smoky hue over red and black houses, and there is an enchanting melody. The human state is recognised by a blue light.

TIBETAN WISDOM

Sonam's master paused, then addressed Nazir. Conversation turned to life in the West. What did we eat in France? Did I have a car? The Rinpoche's curiosity and interest extended from technology, houses and books, education and sport to the price of gold. The two subjects he did not enquire about were religion and medicine. He was enthralled by details of the Paris Metro. I, in turn, wanted to know why he had chosen to be a medical lama.

Before his birth, he said, astrologers had predicted that he would be a Tulku, and at the age of six, at his grandmother's suggestion, the family oracle was asked if the child should be trained in medicine. The oracle, a female deity, communicated through an antique bowl in which were placed marked pieces of paper. When it spun off on its own accord, spilling the answer to the floor, his future calling was confirmed. Since soothsaying was a normal occurrence, I asked why the government in Lhasa had not been more prepared for the Chinese invasion, and why had the people, so attached to spiritual wisdom, had their culture attacked by the full force of communism?

The Rinpoche smiled and sipped his tea before answering. The British invasion in 1904 had been predicted, he said. The coming of the Chinese was also foretold, but few had taken it seriously. Degenerate spiritual values, the misuse of priestly authority and corruption, and the laxity in the monasteries had grown over the centuries to weaken Buddhism. Karma took its toll.

It was destined for people in the West to collect Tibet's wisdom and put it into their own books. 'Soon, no more masters will incarnate. No more teachers. We know this. In the future, people will read about it, but I can not say how they will use the knowledge. We are in the Kali Yuga, the long, long cycle of gathering darkness and materialism. The Buddha will come again, the Buddha Maitreya. We show him standing or sitting in European fashion. It is predicted he will be born in the West.' When and where, the Rinpoche did not say. Study, he advised, since everything we learn in one life is a treasure we guard for the next, to be picked up from where we left off.

In a niche in the wall behind the Tulku, Sonam had put a gilded bronze statue of the Buddha of Medicine. It had not been there on our first visit. The Buddha's right hand falling across his knee, had its palm upwards in the gesture of giving and held a branch in flower. The left hand against the diaphragm held a vase of ambrosia, symbol of longevity. Following my eyes, the Rinpoche took the moment to 'expand our knowledge'.

THE BUDDHA OF MEDICINE

The Buddha of Medicine was there for us to meditate on and to take refuge in his being by visualising his form with all its characteristics, or by looking at an actual statue. In one of the most used rituals, the letter 'OM' is imagined white on his forehead, the letter 'AH', red on his throat, and the letter 'HUNG', sapphire blue on his heart. 'OM' is the germ syllable of all physical attributes of an illuminated being. 'AH', is the verbal qualities and 'HUNG', the mental. The white light of 'OM' enters us through the crown chakra and fills us with the Buddha's living energy. The red ray of 'AH' hits the throat chakra to cleanse our words, and the blue ray of 'HUNG' touches the heart chakra bestowing intuition. Finally, rays of all colours shoot out from the Buddha's seven chakras to unite in our heart. When taking refuge in the Buddha of Medicine, we must ask for his compassion towards every living being.

For the Wind Nopa, one imagined a luminous, warm substance

with the consistency of butter flowing from the Buddha to us and then returning into his form via the head chakra. In the same way, the Bile Nopa was pacified by a light resembling cool water, the Phlegm Nopa corrected by a warm, red light. If the disorder is localised, that area must be touched by the appropriate ray corresponding to the imbalanced Nopa. The ray creates an opening for the subtle vapours to escape, and when the illness is not restricted to a particular area, the vapours are visualised leaving the body via the genitals and anus. At the end, the Buddha's image is dissolved from the outside inwards.

'I assure you these methods, when practised with regular breathing, in, held, and expired, each to the count of six, will revive the system and help to prevent aging', advised the Rinpoche. 'The Tantric anatomy forms a bridge from the spiritual to the physical. The condition of the subtle body and its energies mirrors itself in the material constitution.'

Sonam worked with the Nopa's malfunctions by dealing with their pathological expression. Here, we had been initiated into the practice of healing through contact with the mystical body. Unreal? Where did matter begin and 'non-matter' end? Any tangible object can be broken down to an essence of probabilities, and when all the skins of an onion are removed, nothing remains but the position of our minds in relation to the inspected object or phenomena. Where are we? Where is reality? Physicists and mystics agree that laws governing matter no longer apply in extreme orders of magnitude. Laws are mind-charts illustrating a reality that may not be the ultimate truth. So why ask if the Nopas are real, how can the mystic Fire Element produce an eye, by what power do Shamans manipulate matter, or do mantras work? In the metaphysics of Tibetan medicine, they had mapped the terrain of interrelating principles. Nothing, they claimed, can be completely explained by the intellect alone.

Is this why the Buddha taught that the ultimate liberation was a return to the void, the 'no-thing'? And in contradictory terms worthy of a zen koan, was this ultimate vacuum *the* actuality from which all probabilities are born, not from nothingness, but from a pregnant emptiness? But emptiness remains empty; the children of its womb are illusions. Out of this double negative had arisen the positive attitude of compassion. I found it simpler and more elegant to assume that in the absence of the universe, space and time, there would be an absence of change, smallness and dividedness, but not a nothing. Beneath what we see could exist changelessness, the infinite, the whole, which is a far cry indeed from nothingness.

The master waved Nazir to bring over our tape recorder, and shown the keys, he enjoyed taping our voices for replay. Sonam asked for polaroid photos. The venerable Tulku watched the images develop with a hearty grin. He then left his seat, and with a cat's suppleness, came to each of us in turn, took our faces between his hands, and with a low mantra, pressed his forehead to ours. In the intimacy of that contact I felt the sincerity of his blessing. We left to stumble home under a moonless sky.

HOMEWARD THOUGHTS

'Well! From what I gather after that talk on death', said Nazir, 'I will be rushing down a dark tunnel towards a light, having gone through psychedelic colours as my chakras open with my binary brain blowing its fuses in complete confusion. And, as I lack their built-in imagery, my Bardo might well be a Mercedes garage and my demon a snow plough ready to push me into an avalanche.' He shivered ostentatiously.

'The Rinpoche said we had a higher part of our mind that is there to guide us', I replied.

'I suppose that gives one hope', he sighed. 'In's Allah! I will suddenly slip off a mountain after a glorious expedition; no lingering death for me!' He hesitated, 'But I won't forget what the old boy said about those visualisations for death. He's right. Life should be led so that one is not ashamed of oneself. I want to be proud when Allah calls me.'

'Who will be the figure at the end of your tunnel?'

'Michael or Gabriel. No! Michael and Gabriel. And you?'

'At this period of my life, I think Vishnu the Preserver, the world's most ancient Avatar, the principle of all Saviours who incarnate to balance Shiva's destruction.'

Even in my closeness to Nazir, I kept my secret. When I had stood in the presence of that statue of Vishnu-Venkataswara, I had been so moved as to follow the example of every pilgrim there, and ask for three requests. They had all been fulfilled against great odds. Those who know don't say, and those who speak say too much.

The Tibetans have had centuries of practice in comforting the dying. Few die here in hospitals with tubes and machines keeping them alive. An intern once confided that after he had resuscitated an elderly priest, the man opened his eyes saying. 'Young man, be careful. You have robbed me of my death.'

'Nazir, are you frightened of dying?'

'Must we go into this right now?' came his voice weary in the darkness.

'Yes. Right now's the time, in the dark night, along our unlit path. Tomorrow we'll be into other things.'

I told him that first, the dying person denies death. Anger takes over, then comes a stage of bargaining with God. As denial, anger and bargaining have no result, the next stage of depression evolves into acceptance.

'And what can be done in practical terms, I mean, to help the dying, and those around him?' asked Nazir walking at a brisk pace without a cigarette for a change.

'Get into contact, let them discuss their fears. Bring the subject into the open, and if they don't have any particular faith, ask what the highlights of their life were, and what for them, is the meaning of existence. The answers are not the most important thing. Sonam gave us the essence. The dying need love. It's far stronger than words and often more difficult to offer.'

'I think one of the problems is that most of us don't want to be enlightened in the Rinpoche's sense. It's too hard and needs such effort. The majority of us would rather pass from one dream here to another somewhere else, hopefully without nightmares in between. That is if you believe in an afterlife. And, if we just want to float off into God knows what, we hope relief from further responsibility will come through oblivion.'

'I'm certain, Nazir, you'll find yourself in a Moslem paradise complete with a Mercedes.'

'And you?'

'Me? I hope to fly off behind the moon and beyond the stars to Apollo's gardens of the sun.'

In the Tibetan Book of the Dead, life and death are approached as six Bardos, or Great Transitions. The three Bardos of Life are earthly existence, the state of sleep and dreams and the meditative experience. Those of death, concern the nature of the mind and its projections, beautiful and terrible which appear to have an objective reality. The texts teach how to understand the origin of these seductive and terrifying visions.

After dinner, I snuggled down. The night's low mist encircled the camp, and I had the odd sensation of existing in a very small place. To make that space safe, I recited an ancient prayer:

From ghoulies and ghosties
and long legged beasties
and things that go bump in the night
Good Lord deliver us!
And may we sleep in peace.

EPILOGUE

———— • ————

Our final meeting with the Amchi—
Perspectives on Tibetan medicine—My return
through Kashmir to Paris—where a
premonition is justified

A FAREWELL PARTY

'Morning!' barked Nazir, raising the tent flap to thrust in an arm
with a mug of tea. I dressed lethargically and crawled out into
the air smelling of damp earth. Departure was scheduled for the
afternoon. This time we would be seeing the landscape in reverse
order. It reminded me of a discipline the monks followed by review-
ing the day's events as if watching a film run backwards. First
efforts invariably drown one in sleep before the process is completed; not the object of an exercise designed for perfect recall.

Nazir hummed and shaved. Gulam and Mohamet made breakfast. They had already put our provisions in a depressing pile for
the trek back to Padum. Nazir and I carefully avoided all mention
of our time in Karsha now about to end. Our mood lightened
considerably the instant we saw Thelmy come galloping bareback
into camp. He jumped off his pony and scuttled over to Nazir.
Sonam's emissary was given fried eggs and chapattis eaten with
his fingers, and in half swallowed sentences he delivered his
uncle's message. We were invited for a farewell gathering in the
Amchi's house at noon. Thelmy, back on his mount, gave it a
series of hard kicks and trotted away singing at the top of his
voice. I could have kidnapped that imp of a sorcerer's apprentice.

I didn't want to pack. Leaving Sonam was an unhappy prospect
after our adoption into his world and the generosity of his instruction. When the midday shadows made dark puddles at our feet,
we set out on our last walk to Sonam's white house. He stood

at the gate to usher us into a cluttered cellar on the ground floor. It was his pharmacy, ordered in its fashion with jars and tins stacked on shelves and sacks hanging from the ceiling. He reached into the corner above a bunch of herbs and pulled down a scroll wrapped in leather. Outside under a tree, he proudly unrolled it for us to admire. On the parchment were front and back views of an androgynous figure spotted with the points of moxabustion. The illustrations, brown with age, were a two-hundred-year-old family heirloom painted by an ancestor, some of whose medical notes were also in Sonam's possession.

He asked for photos of the diagram, and to our amazement, added the request of a thermometer. Apart from his praise for western surgery, he had shown scant interest in our technology, and, in fact, had no real need for an instrument to measure the body's heat, so expertly assessed through the pulses. The thermometer, he explained, a little abashed, was to intrigue his patients and accustom them to modern, foreign methods. 'We have to learn more about each other's ways', he said.

We promised to dispatch the thermometer from Srinagar. He grinned, in his expression a hint of doubt, if not of our intentions, then in their execution. Then, withdrawing a stone and a packet of pills from the inner pocket of his robe, he pressed them into my hand. The small, green stone was to be bound for ten minutes, wrapped in a cloth impregnated with hot oil, on a point below the ankle bone. That, and the herbal pills would help but not cure my eyes. There wasn't time to supervise a long cure. Sonam required at least six months. I needed *ukpa*, and various other herbal compounds and distillations which he could not prepare because they would have to be adjusted in response to my reactions. His gifts, given freely, were, he said, like our aspirins. They might alleviate, but not cure my allergy.

We asked what we might do for him. He turned away, clapped his hands and shouted up to the window of his room. His sister, her two children, Pema from the monastery and his elder brother, the school teacher, came rushing down the stairs. Thelmy brought up the rear. Dressed in their best, the children's noses wiped, they gathered around the Amchi. No! It was not right. They broke away shouting in excitement to dash off behind the house.

A piercing whinny announced the arrival of Sonam's stallion, bridled and saddled for his master. He mounted, and centred in his rightful place above them all, he posed for family portraits. Their expressions changed from remote seriousness to sheer glee as they watched the polaroids develop in their hands.

In Sonam's room, the table, laid with a white cloth under cups, the usual kettle replaced by a china tea pot next to a red thermos made in China, the cakes and flowers, showed the trouble taken to make our final gathering a celebration prepared so carefully despite the adults having worked in the fields since dawn.

We sat ready for high conversation. None came. We smiled at each other, sipped tea and munched ginger biscuits and rice cakes, making exaggerated noises of appreciation. We were all very self-conscious. It was no relief when the Amchi's sister enquired about our health; had we enjoyed our stay? Have another cake? Did we require food for our journey? Her questions seemed interminable, and our intensely polite replies did nothing to cheer up the deteriorating situation that we could see was becoming an embarrassment for all present. Most notably the Amchi whose unusual lack of composure was registered in light grunts between mouthfuls of scalding tea.

'My God! I can't take much more of this', mumbled Nazir between translations, 'I've a feeling they all have work to do but don't know how to end our visit without appearing abrupt and at the same time quite sincerely wanting to give us a fine send off. So, I'm going to say; Amchi-man, you're great. We thank you, so let's get out the chang and have some fun.' Sonam's head went back in a great laugh. He reached under the bed to pull out a stone jar of chang, and the atmosphere of stiffling restraint that had covered our real feeling lifted in a spate of toasts, five in a row; to our abundant prosperity, to theirs, each of us wished the others good health, and for future happiness we drank overfilled glasses to our return and may our footsteps never stray from the Buddha's path.

'Just remember to send me more photos, please,' said Sonam as he shook our hands. We filed from the room, my nose tingling with the aroma of dried herbs. In time to come, whenever I encountered that smell, it evoked Sonam, the family, the valley, the wind, and the dust.

TIBETAN MEDICINE

In Sonam's medicine, every aspect of life is given value. Their creed copes with the polarity of body and spirit. The opposition of gods and demons offers a coherent psychology for both disease

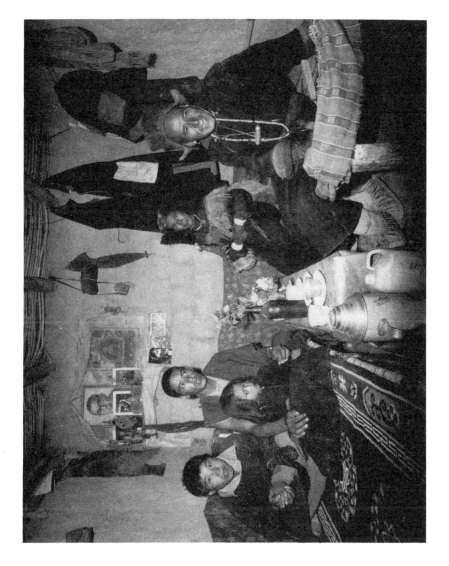

Family gathering (from left to right) Thelmy (pulling a face), Pema with one of his nieces, Sonam's sister Dolka and Sonam and healing – it is their powers that heal or afflict. More important than the obscurities and contradictions in their metaphysics, the Dharma's teachings make sense to all Tibetans and Ladakhis. They understand the measure of their own individual and karmic responsibility in falling sick and cultivate a positive response in both behaviour and prayers for recovery. Cultural ties between doctor and patient pave the way for a relationship of mutual concern and trust.

A highly refined method of diagnosis covers the pathological and the psychological sides of illness always logically defined. The devotion of qualified Amchis and medical priests alike exemplify the Buddha's way. The very depth of their wisdom throws into relief the charlatanism of others less fortunate in their knowledge, but who, in the words of Marco Polo, are prepared to sport with the blindness of deluded and wretched people. Yet the people of the Zangskar, if deluded in their superstitions, are far from wretched. Their unabashed love of life coupled to humour and the sense of belonging to a close-knit Buddhist society, lifts even the poorest from despair. Sonam's request for a thermometer, indicated the intrusion of new ideas into an established tradition that was already well oriented to dispel ignorance.

A SAD FAREWELL

Bags packed, rubbish buried and light luggage slung over our shoulders, when we saw Sonam on the goat path, we expected only a short round of handshakes before we left. But he insisted on helping to carry our things to the river where the ferrymen waited with their perilous rubber dinghy.

The men, up to their knees in water, fiddled about checking for leaks. Above the steep banks on the far side, the plateau stretched to Padum. Along its edge billowed a yellow cloud. Miracle! We would actually have some transport; a cart pulled by a tractor. Nazir let out a whoop. Sonam clapped and thumped Nazir on the back and pushed him off on the first crossing to flag down the driver chugging over the flats.

I stayed next to Sonam. Aware of the significance of this time of transition, my attention nevertheless wandered, and I gazed dumbly at the wild land, its outlines softened under a sky sucked white with wind. It was no diversion from heartache. On the dinghy's return, just as I was about to step in, Sonam drew me

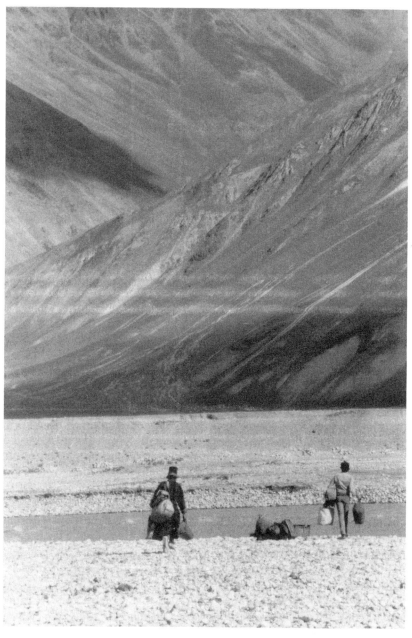

Sonam helps with the luggage on our last day together

aside. Without a word, he fastened round my neck a short coral necklace. His eyes glistened. When we shoved off in the swirl, I waved and shouted my adieu. The sound, absorbed into the air and the rush of water, became symbolic of change itself. We had joined him to live in the body of our shared experiences. Now that body was dying; its components were being separated and released.

Sonam remained at the river's edge, an hieratic figure with one arm raised in salute, and alone, behind him the mountain. He grew smaller and smaller as the ferrymen paddled me across the water in the first lap towards another world so very far away. We left Sonam in a terrain where his senses are in harmony with nature's changing moods. The winds of life blow through his philosophy, and rest in his being. He rides from one impoverished village to another, where with compassion and humour he combats delusion. Without extravagance there is no generosity; without generosity there is no love, without love no understanding. He is the Amchi.

In our last look from the plateau, Nazir said, 'Sonam will always be there, standing at the gateway to our dreams.'

RETURN JOURNEY

The tractor driver had been persuaded to carry us to Padum for a few rupees, and settled in the cart we clattered over ground, belching trails of dust. Packs of children ran from the fields and hamlets to yelp and wave, but the scamps had none of the charm of our young Karsha shepherds. The sun sank as we trundled into the school yard occupied by three trekkers in blue and orange tents. Alongside the building the lorries were parked, ready for the convoy next day.

In the cold pre-dawn, we rose for departure with the trekkers. Today, they have a mobility and lightness of equipment, whereas a hundred years ago an adventurer in Ladakh required a large caravan of beasts and porters. The 260 miles between Srinagar and Leh took nineteen days, and bearing a load for a single European could easily involve fourteen coolies. Yet, accounts written in the early 1900s have not dated and descriptions of people and scenery and customs are as recognisable now as they were in the past.

At 5am sharp, the lorries pulled out. It would be a fast journey in empty vehicles, a one day ride. We dozed intermittently, jarred

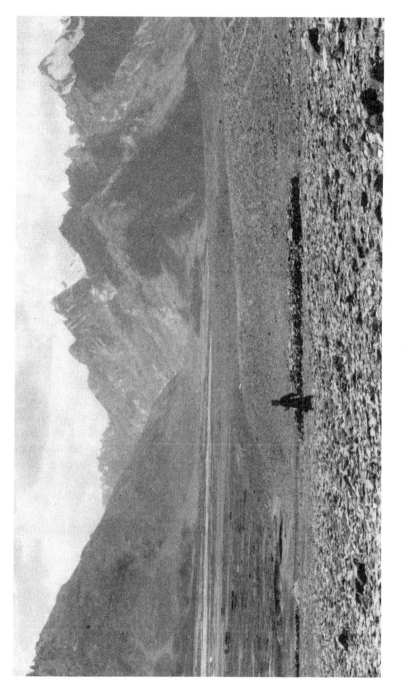

Sonam strides through his domain

from slumber by bumps and choked by flurries of dust. Late that afternoon, I caught a glimpse of a Ladakhi family herding their horses back into the Zangskar. The troop trotted by. One woman wore incongruous dark glasses under her parak. The scene gave me a fit of nostalgia for what we had left, and the image remained with me more vivid and poignant than any photograph.

The peaks of Nun and Kun ablaze in the sunset marked the end of the Buddha's domain and the point where the minarets of Islam rose to grace the hamlets. Grey with fatigue and dust, after seventeen hours we staggered from the lorry, heads light, and with stiff legs walked into Kargil's only open restaurant for plates of soggy rice and volcanic mutton curry.

Next morning, I felt like a clock with a broken spring. Exciting times had run down into boredom. An hour and a half went by before Nazir roared down the main street in his jeep, hooter honking for Gulam and Mohamet to load up. We left Kargil with no second thoughts, and the old joy returned. We were on the move, this time in our own vehicle and on a road, that after the Zangskar, had a right to call itself a highway. Back to Sonamarg, and on, down to the rice fields, ripened and bathed in the colours softened by moist air. Wind-battered and drowsy, we drove into Abdul's garden in time to hear the last call from the mosque.

In the peace of the houseboats moored under the chenar trees by the lake, attention to our every need gave us three days of luxury, and time to assimilate my experiences. Life had softness by the lake, an atmosphere far removed from the Amchi's world. Propped up on my elbow in the houseboat, I looked out on a carpet of waterlily leaves splattered with drops of rain transformed into moonstones with a brilliance that lasted until their loveliness was drunk by the sun. Just so, many of our thoughts evaporate before they come to fruition, floating in the ether unattached to action.

In the evenings, Nazir paddled the shikara, and when he sang, I was transported beyond the lake, above the mountains, back to the deserts of Ladakh. On the day of my departure a biting wind blew off the autumn snow cloaking the Srinagar hills. Purple clouds brushed their summits. 'It's never the right time to leave, is it?' said Nazir, 'but summer is dead and another will come and another and you will return to us. In's Allah!' he concluded with a wry grin.

Delhi, Kabul and a diversion via Moscow brought me back to Paris. On entering the apartment after an absence in an elemental land blessed with space, the living room, with all its associations seemed smaller. I saw each object with a renewed appreciation, and memories that fluttered about their shapes no longer upset me. There was no need to chase them away. They had their place and were, as I had come to understand, necessary ingredients of life. Sonam had spoken of post-digestive change in the qualities of an ingredient, and something of the sort had happened in the alchemy of my mind.

Although my eyes remained uncured, my sojourn with Sonam had healed me of a far greater discomfort. That part of me trapped in the past was now free. It had been a continuous process, sometimes obscure, sometimes obvious like, for instance, the night after dancing below Karsha monastery when rememberances had ceased to trouble my heart; that moment of wholeness on my return from the Lha-mo; or the hour I had parted from Sonam leaving him to his world where in the mirror of their foreign ways I had learnt more than facts about Tibetan medicine and now saw myself more clearly. I had no definite answers to anything, just a few clues to throw light on a human enigma.

On my desk a pile of mail spilt over the 'I Ching', the Book of Changes. A black rimmed card announced Alice's death. She had died on the very morning I had sensed her release, and in the following time of grief and happiness, of loss and gain, the Amchi strode into my mind. His presence was there and I recalled his words in the lamp-lit kitchen, for we are all linked to the pulses of those we love.

APPENDIX 1

---·---

BUDDHISM AND TIBETAN MEDICINE

Closely linked with Buddhism, Tibetan medicine is based on the 3500 year old Vedic scriptures of India, the same tradition into which the Buddha himself was born in 563 BC. The Brahmins classify existence into two spheres, the spiritual and the material. Man stands in between, partaking of both. The Five Elements, Fire, Earth, Air, Water and Space, are the principles of life that give it substance. They act both in man and throughout the universe as a whole. In harmony they cause well-being; in discord they cause illness.

From Brahminic observations and logic came the framework for a rational science in which medicine had its role. While medical investigation and therapy progressed, theory hardly evolved at all. Anatomical functions, ruled by subtle energy, made the tangible subservient to the spiritual, and priest/doctors attempting to keep the forces of life in balance, stressed the importance of thought, behaviour and diet in health.

The idea of reincarnation was already well-established when the Buddha was born. Man's acts determined his destiny. In the course of his evolution his consciousness returns time after time to an earthly body trapped in a world of illusion from which, ultimately purified and enlightened, the Atman or eternal spirit of the Hindu, will be absorbed into that unity that lies beyond all creation.

The Buddha, commenting on the suffering that comes from incarnation, said 'I teach of pain and the cessation of pain'. The ultimate cause of suffering is ignorance. Harmony, health and the end of suffering come from devotion to the Buddha's way. To the Buddhist, medicine, the art of healing both the mind and the body, has never been divorced from religious practice. Many in the west pay lip service to this holistic approach to life. Few of us make the commitment on a material and a spiritual level that will ensure its success.

APPENDIX 2

———————— • ————————

THE THREE NOPAS

Tibetan medicine is founded on the theory of the Three Nopas. Their disposition and qualities, their functions, especially in digestion and their workings on health and sickness hardly differ from those of their Ayurvedic origins in India. This ancient concept of the three Humours also travelled into classical Greece, and from there to the Mediterranean and Medieval Europe.

The concept of the five Elements and the Three Nopas came to Tibet from Vedic philosophy. The predominance of one reveals the individual's general constitution and denotes a particular physical type and its pathological disposition. Influenced by the seasons, the Nopas rise and fall in very much the same way as biorhythms. The Wind Nopa peaks in the Autumn, Bile in Winter and Phlegm in Spring.

Classification of disease, diet, medicine and therapy correspond to the dominant Nopa's inherent nature that generates physiological function while maintaining its own subtle activity. The Nopa upholds the body's seven main constituents formed by its digestive action.

Each constituent arises from the essence of the one that precedes it in a week-long metabolic cycle. First is chyle, the essence of which produces blood, flesh, fat, bone marrow, seminal fluids and menstrual flow. When a Nopa's power is out of balance, it augments, diminishes or upsets the activity in its own specific area and consequently the seven constituents that it controls.

The Nopas could be seen as a very loose analogy to the development of the early human embryo. Its inside layer grows into the stomach and lungs. Its middle layer into bones, muscles and blood vessels. Its outer layer into skin and the nervous system. Some psychiatrists believe that a predominance of one of these layers can predispose the character of an individual as digestive, muscular or cerebral. The subtle anatomy of the mystic body consists of three main channels. On the right hand side of the spine runs the 'Ro-ma'. It is connected to the hot, red principle and is linked with the sun, the Element of Fire and the Bile Nopa. The Ro-ma induces the formation of the vascular system.

The 'Kyang-ma' channel runs on the left hand side of the spine. It is related to the cool, white principle and is associated with the moon, the Elements of Water and Earth, and the Phlegm Nopa. It brings into existence semen, nerves, tendons and the brain.

Uniting these two antagonistic types of energy is the central channel of the Bu-ma. Neutral in principle, the Bu-ma is associated with the Elements of Air and Aether. Its Nopa, the Wind, brings into being the genital organs.

The right and central channels meet at the base of the heart where they unite blood (Bile Nopa) with air (Wind Nopa). The Seven Chakras, of which five are used in medicine and two in meditation, are located on the central Bu-ma. They ascend from a point between the genitals and the anus to the crown of the head.

APPENDIX 3

---•---

THE MONASTERY AT KARSHA

Founded in the fifteenth century the monastery at Karsha is the most illustrious in the Zangskar and one of the four principal seats of the reformed Gelugpa or 'Yellow Hat' order, headed by the Dalai Lama. Over 160 monks live in the monastery itself. The monastery owns over 200 acres of land and thirteen villages. Another thirteen villages in the area are affiliated to the older sects of the 'Red Hat' or Nyngmapa order.

Boys of six are taken in for four years of study and oral examination. Then, if they wish, they can become part of the religious community. After twelve years on probation they will take the 253 monastic vows that precede ordination. A novice is seldom younger than 20 years of age. No perpetual vows exist. Monks are free to leave at any time. In the course of training, according to seniority and merit, they are invested with special functions such as conducting rites and liturgies, organising sacred dances or performing extra mural activities.

One of the highest positions in the hierarchy is that of the Abbot. He has a dual function as spiritual director and head of education. Monks become doctors of philosophy, theology or medicine, but there is a clear distinction drawn between purely scholastic knowledge and wisdom in the gnostic sense. Nuns, deprived of the same opportunities are little more than peasants. They pray and work the monastery's lands.

APPENDIX 4

---•---

Although Indian law banned polyandry in 1948, in most parts of Ladakh, the custom still persists. Introduced in the eighteenth century, it is an effective way of limiting births in an austere and harsh environment. A woman shared between two brothers can lead to as much jealousy as a man shared between two sisters. But if she should inherit, she is free to pick her own husband, does not have to share her wealth with him and if he displeases her, can, at a moment's notice, send him packing.

Unmarried women are left with few options unless they are educated. They can become nuns, servants or army prostitutes, a profession unknown before the early sixties when Leh became a garrison town after the Sino-Indian war. Although love matches are increasingly popular among the urban young, most marriages are arranged. An astrologer computes the compatibility of the future couple and the two families remain in close contact before and after the wedding.

In a society officially without castes, three main socio-economic groups continue to be recognised. The nobility keep very much to themselves although they occasionally marry Moslems or Christians. The second category includes artists, artisans, farmers, some merchants and shepherds. Woe betide a woman from either of the two higher classes who marries a blacksmith, musician or beggar: she joins the outcasts.

Women are never idle, they spin the wool that men weave and are seldom at a loss in speaking their minds or giving advice. Today, Ladakh's 1000 year old royal dynasty is represented by the political leader, Queen Deskit Wangmo, who has a seat in the Indian parliament. She has plans to exploit the country's virtually untouched mineral resources, build hydro electric dams and generally encourage progress for a people with one foot firmly planted in the past and the other ready for a blue-jeaned future.

For centuries, Ladakhi communities have been guided by monks in their world of study, meditation, ceremony and identification with the immortal. Wars and famine, the injustice or generosity of men have been accepted and endured as events endemic in a world of precarious fortune. But today, there are also women aware of change who have a growing sense of social obligation. Guardians of their national culture, they travel the land to advise on child care, encourage monogamy and drum up political support for young Buddhist activists in an effort to preserve traditions threatened by Indian administration and Moslem economic expansion.